VLADIMIR TULINOV

THE GUARDSMEN OF HIPPOCRATES

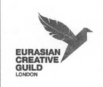

EURASIAN
CREATIVE
GUILD
LONDON

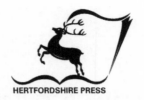

HERTFORDSHIRE PRESS

Printed in United Kingdom
Cambridge International Press
Imprint of Hertfordshire Press Ltd © 2019
e-mail: publisher@hertfordshirepress.com
www.hertfordshirepress.com

On behalf of Eurasian Creative Guild, London

EURASIAN
CREATIVE
GUILD
LONDON

THE GUARDSMEN OF HIPPOCRATES
by VLADIMIR TULINOV ©

English

Edited by Jesse Alexander
Typeset by Alexandra Rey

British Library Catalogue in Publication Data
A catalogue record for this book is available from the British Library
Library of Congress in Publication Data
A catalogue record for this book has been requested

ISBN: 978-1-910886-94-6

CONTENTS

THE RED CROSS

One in four soldiers has already been killed.
Stretching on the white-red snow,
 A girl is alone on the battle field.
 She pants:'I must do it, must go!'
But the man is too heavy for dragging,
I'll never keep hold.'
(The nurse is too weak for pulling,
She is only eighteen years old).

Yulia Drunina

The battalion duty sergeant, a tall man with an armband on the left sleeve of his faded and mended tunic, tried to get to the point of the travel order, which Tatyana had taken out of her breast pocket. But he couldn't focus on reading the document.

Having glanced at the sly eyes of the beautiful woman standing in front of him, the sergeant rubbed his crimson cheeks, folded the paper in four and picked up Tanya's1 rucksack. Then he led the fair-haired girl on, moving fast along the narrow, winding trench.

---

1   *Tanya is a familiar form of Tatyana. Russian first names have several forms depending on the level of formality in a given situation.*

In the dugout, to the right of the entrance, stood a metal stove. A little farther on the right there were two tiers of four rough bunks. In the centre stood something like a table, covered with a piece of long canvas which hung down to the earthen floor. On the table there was a field telephone, a night light, an ashtray, and some papers. Near the left wall stood a bench and two upturned metal barrels. In the corner there was a safe, shelves, and something else which was hardly visible in the twilight.

The battalion commander, a lean brown-haired man of about thirty-five, finished his conversation and absent-mindedly fidgeted with Tanya's travel order. Having thrown it on the table, he suddenly shouted into the receiver, 'When will you send dogs? You've been promising for two months! Could you at least send two teams?'

Tanya was startled, and asked 'What do they need dogs for here? In teams!?'

It was obvious that the answer about the dogs didn't satisfy the commander. Hitting the telephone receiver in annoyance, he angrily said to the black-haired officer, 'Pavlenko is all talk and no action! I'll report him to the regimental commander.'

After pouring tea from the small kettle standing on the stove into a tin mug, the commander of the battalion took a few sips and turned to the girl, saying with a frown, 'I'm Miroshnikov, the battalion commander, and the man who is sitting at the table is the executive officer, Captain Pichkhadze. The head physician of the regiment told me about you by telephone. I know you want to be a medical instructor in the company.'

The commander shook his head and carefully looked at the slim girl and her close-fitting new uniform.

'How much do you weigh?' he asked. His unexpected question hung in the air.

The executive officer left his papers and with eyes, tired of insomnia, stared at the thin, stubble-covered face of the commander.

'I d-don't know,' murmured Tanya. 'I was last weighed long ago.'

'Well I know!' Miroshnikov said sharply.

Getting up from the stool, he lowered his head to avoid the log ceiling of the dugout, and, taking a step towards the girl, said in a cool voice, 'You weigh three and a half puds,[2] Tatyana Rusakova – not more. That's why you are not fit for being a medic. A soldier doesn't go over the top in his drawers, but in uniform, with weapons and equipment. All that weighs about eighty kilos. And those kilograms are to be dragged off the battlefield quickly, with the rifle, by the way. How will you manage to do that?'

'I'll manage, Comrade Major!'

The girl's voice sounded so firm and resolute, that the commander stopped talking, waved his hand in disappointment and, taking a seat on a bunk in the corner of the small dugout, began to roll a cigarette.

The silence was broken by the dark-haired executive officer.

'You insist on being sent to the front, Comrade Rusakova. Praiseworthy indeed, but you can't imagine what

2   *A historical measure of weight (also **pood**) which is equal to nearly 36 lbs (16.3 kg).*

it means. In the regimental medical centre the medical staff live in tents. Our men equipped two dugouts for doctors and nurses. While in rifle companies at the front line all personnel have equal conveniences – foxholes and trenches. The commander is giving you sensible advice. I know that before the war you studied midwifery. To deliver a baby is one thing, and to pull a wounded soldier from the battlefield another...'

The telephone rang, and the executive officer picked up the receiver. As he listened to whomever was on the other end of the line, red blotches gradually appeared on his face. After answering a curt 'We'll give the command soon, just wait,' the officer turned to the battalion commander and said, 'Not good. First Lieutenant Zhelnov reports that in the dugout in No Man's Land, he has six badly wounded soldiers bleeding profusely. The machine gunner, Second Sergeant Timokhin, managed to crawl to the company trench line despite wounds in both legs. The six soldiers stayed in the dugout, and the medical instructor was killed in the afternoon during a fascist attack.'

'Alright, Guram,' Miroshnikov addressed the executive officer by name, as he did when he was excited. "Send medical assistant Sayenko quickly and–'

'Sayenko is wounded, Comrade Major, by a shell fragment,' the executive officer clarified hurriedly. 'He bandaged himself and continued to help the wounded, but eventually lost consciousness. An hour ago, he was sent to the regimental aid station on a medical cart.'

Gritting his teeth, the commander turned to the girl, who was standing at attention. 'First, rest. Second,

I appoint you medical instructor in the first company.' Miroshnikov raised his voice upon seeing the girl's eyes light up, 'Temporarily, for one day: to be exact, for one night.'

The commander put out his cigarette and threw it into the ashtray, an artillery shell casing which had been cut in half. Looking at Tatyana, he said in a tired voice: 'In the early morning the Germans attacked, five times. And we began to counterattack. Just before your arrival the fascists calmed down. The fighting was heavy, there were many killed and wounded men. More than a hundred soldiers were sent to the regimental medical centre, and that's not the end of it. In half an hour it will be dark. The medical orderlies will begin to mop up the front line. Usually after fighting like that about thirty wounded soldiers are found.'

The officer stopped talking, glanced at the clock, lifted the receiver and put it down again. He addressed the girl, but not according to regulations. 'Go to First Company's location with Sedoy, who is with Medical Assistant Maltsev. There you'll be told what to do.'

'Comrade Major!' Pichkhadze cried and jumped up from the table. 'The best medical assistant?! We have sixteen wounded soldiers at the battalion medical centre, and at night more will be brought in.'

'They will bring and send them as ordered!' Miroshnikov said angrily. 'In the medical centre we have the platoon commander, the medical assistant, and his orderlies. They will do the job. And in the dugout, there are six badly wounded soldiers. We need Maltsev to get them to us alive.'

The executive officer nodded and, dialing the phone, began to give short orders. The battalion commander addressed the girl: 'You are at the disposal of Sergeant Maltsev. Try to remember everything he does and says. You'll need it many times in the future.'

Miroshnikov took the knife that was lying on the barrel, turned it upside down and opened a tin of fish. Then he poured strong tea into a tin mug from the pot that stood on the stove. Picking up a dry crust of black bread, he invited the newly-minted medical instructor to have supper. 'Stuff yourself, and that's an order!' he joked, cutting off her attempt to refuse the invitation. 'You'll have a hard night, so take a seat and get some energy into you.'

Tanya, who hadn't had a crumb in her mouth since morning, sat down on the edge of the bunk and tucked heartily into the plain fare, casting a grateful glance at Miroshnikov's grey, insomniac features.

A broad-shouldered man in a greatcoat pulled the canvas aside, bent his head and dove into the dugout. 'Comrade Major, Sergeant Maltsev reporting as ordered,' Maltsev saluted crisply.

'Did the executive officer explain the mission to you?' the commander asked quietly.

'Yes, just now, over the telephone.'

'Take everything you need from the battalion medical centre. Zhelnov will send stretcher-bearers. The medical instructor will help you. She arrived today.' Miroshnikov pointed at Tanya, who was wiping crumbs from the table. 'Find a greatcoat for her. That's all. Do it!'

Stars were twinkling here and there in the gaps in the cloudy sky, and the sickle-shaped moon seemed to be playing hide and seek with them. It disappeared behind a quick-moving cloud and then re-appeared for a moment to touch the ground with a narrow wisp of cold light.

Tanya huddled up. The impudent wind got under her skirt, tried to knock her cap off, ruffled her hair, and turned her uniform's tunic into a sail.

'Take mine for a while,' said the sergeant, who was the first to leave the dugout, as he put his greatcoat around her shoulders. 'Wait for me here and don't leave the dugout.'

The greatcoat had been warmed by the body of the broad-shouldered doctor's assistant, and Tanya felt warm. To keep from losing it in the wind, she squatted in the dugout and leaned against the wall.

'He is caring!' Tanya thought with delight about the sergeant. She also noticed that his face was young, and his temples were for some reason grey.

The sergeant came back faster than one could imagine.

'Take the medic bag and the kit, and I'll carry the rest,' he ordered in a low voice and put on his greatcoat. Looking into the eyes of the girl, he gave brief instructions: 'In the trenches, follow me. We'll bend down while crossing exposed terrain. Don't lose sight of me. We are short of time, and it's not less than a kilometre from here to the positions of the first company.'

He pulled his cap down over his forehead and picked up two heavy, oval things that looked like suitcases. He moved along the trench, leading towards the forest, which could hardly be seen in the enveloping darkness.

'Hold on, Tanyukha!' Tanya encouraged herself as she followed the sergeant. Biting her lip, she struggled not to lose sight of the doctor's assistant hurrying ahead. Suddenly his figure appeared right in front of her, her nose a hair's breadth from his back.

'We are leaving the trench now,' the sergeant whispered. 'We'll cross the field to the wood with short dashes. If the Germans begin to fire tracers, we crawl. If there is a flare, we stay still. Got it?'

Tanya nodded in agreement. She was beginning to like the sergeant.

'He is experienced,' she thought with respect. 'He must have been at the front for a long time.'

'I think it will be quiet,' the doctor's assistant said, perhaps wishing to encourage his companion. 'The Germans are licking their wounds after their Pyrrhic victory.'

'Victory?'

'They advanced and drove back the company to the edge of the forest. They thought they had won. But our soldiers summoned up their strength and rushed to counterattack. They beat them severely. So, the fascists went back to their starting position.'

It took them nearly half an hour to get to the company. Two thick spruce trees, felled by explosions one on top of the other, gave some shelter. Behind them there was a fresh pit, covered with a canvas roof of sorts fixed in place with small sticks.

Lighting the faces of the newcomers with a pocket lantern, the commander of the company, a red-haired, broad-faced officer, shook the hand of the doctor's assistant and nodded to Tatyana. Then he adjusted a dirty neck bandage and said gloomily, 'We have no medical orderlies. Two were killed outright, two more were badly wounded and sent to the battalion aid post. I'll allocate stretcher-bearers to help you – but only four, I can't send more. Losses are very heavy. Oh mother, dear! My heroic warriors fought all day, nevertheless they must still protect the company perimeter. The three platoon commanders were killed, and the First Sergeant was wounded. This is the situation.'

Addressing Maltsev, he added in a begging tone, 'Listen to me, Sedoy. My political instructor is in that dugout. His name is Zhenya Bystrov. Earlier, he took the rest of the company and counterattacked. But for him... do what you can.'

'I understand, Comrade Senior Lieutenant. Permission to leave?'

The sergeant saluted and helped Tatyana out of the pit. Nearby, four soldiers of the company were waiting for them. The hands of two soldiers were busy with rolled canvas stretchers.

'And where are the stakes?' asked Maltsev, looking at the bearers' equipment.

'Here they are on the stretchers, Comrade Sergeant, there are ten stakes of different lengths,' one of the soldiers said in a low voice.

'Take the canteens and the kit bag from the medical instructor,' the doctor's assistant ordered. 'But be careful. Try not to tip them over when you have to crawl.'

Hunched over, the group moved one by one to the edge of the front, the trenches of the company strong points. The wind had died away in the meantime. The rare clouds in the sky did not prevent the moon from standing out in all its beauty in the company of numerous stars that had thickly covered the sky.

'Private Mishin and his friend will take you to the dugout,' a stocky soldier in a greatcoat, torn on one side, told Maltsev, who had jumped into the machinegun pit. 'It is some four hundred metres from here.'

Mishin's "friend" was a small thin dog of unknown breed. Straining at its leash, it led the group of soldiers, headed by the doctor's assistant, into the darkness.

The soldiers followed the guide in single file. Suddenly, the silence was broken by the rattle of an enemy machine gun and the darkness was cut by crimson bolts of fire. The soldiers clung to the ground.

'The German machine guns are using tracer bullets,' the doctor's assistant explained to Tanya, who was lying nearby. Waiting for a pause in the death-dealing fireworks, he ordered quietly, 'Keep on crawling!'

The dog also crawled along near the guide and carried out the order. Suddenly it stopped, and, smelling the air, pulled the leash sharply to the right.

'What did it smell, Mishin?' Maltsev asked anxiously. 'A mine?'

The guide shook his head. 'No, I think that is one of our soldiers, maybe a German.'

'Wounded?'

'We'll find out soon.'

The dog returned to the guide, and, wagging its tail, pulled the leash towards the dugout.

'A dead man is lying there,' Mishin announced, 'We must mark the place.'

'Are you sure?' Maltsev asked doubtfully.

'Alma is never wrong,' the guide responded confidently.

The doctor's assistant took some white cloth out of the kit, tore off a piece and gave it to the bearer. The soldier took a stake from the stretchers, disappeared into the darkness, but came back a minute later. Returning the cloth and the stake, he spat, 'There's a dead German lying there. I couldn't find his rifle, but there was a grenade on his belt. We'll use it.'

The harassing fire from the German side forced the group to crawl the rest of the way across the field, which was pocked with shell holes. Alma veered off course a few times and found bodies of soldiers of the first company and their enemies, German infantrymen. The soldiers, alive just a few hours ago, now lay breathless. Some of them died defending their Motherland, the others died invading a foreign country.

The dugout and the entrance to it were disguised so carefully, that without a four-legged friend it would have been impossible to find. The entrance to the dugout was blocked by the body of a fallen soldier. Seemingly, death had caught him at the very moment he was trying to get into the shelter.

'It's Danilov, the company medical instructor,' the guide whispered, pulling the slain man from the entrance.

'He has a wound in the back of the head. Shrapnel,' Maltsev whispered after examining the dead soldier's head with a small lantern partially wrapped in gauze. 'He was killed on the spot.'

In the dugout, the doctor's assistant hid the gauze in the pocket of his greatcoat, and the lantern filled the gloomy space with its pale light. The wounded lay on the bunks and on the earthen floor lay. Someone was groaning and asking for a drink. A soldier with a bandaged head in the corner was delirious and tried to get up from the bed. The smell of blood, urine, and medicine filled the air in the dugout with a vile-smelling mixture.

'I and the medical instructor will work inside,' Maltsev said as he opened the doors of the dugout wide and ordered, 'Everyone else stay nearby and watch the situation carefully. Only come inside if I call you.'

The sergeant noticed three cubes on the collar of the wounded man lying at the entrance. 'This is the political instructor of the company, Bystrov,' Maltsev turned to Tanya, who was standing behind his back. 'Judging by his breathing, it is a pneumothorax.3 Quickly, take off his tunic and undershirt.' Upon removing the greatcoat, Maltsev hung the lantern from the ceiling and opened the medical bag.

'Comrade Sergeant,' Tanya said quietly, 'the bandage is soaked through with blood and needs to be replaced. Blood and foam are running from the wound.'

'It's an open pneumothorax,' said Maltsev, as soon as he glanced at the wound. 'Give me a wound dressing, quickly!'

---

3   *Commonly referred to as a collapsed lung.*

Tanya took a packed dressing out of the medical kit and held it out to the sergeant. Maltsev threw the old bandage on the floor, tore the packet a little, cleaned the area round the wound with iodine for a few seconds, and put a gauze tampon on the bloody perforation.

'He's a real magician!' Tanya thought while watching the quick movements of the doctor's hands.

'The chest is asymmetrical. The left lung isn't working, the air is in the pleural cavity,' the doctor's assistant concluded confidently.

Maltsev unfolded the rubberized cover of the packet, put it on the wound and began to bandage it. Carefully supporting the wounded man's back, Tanya helped the doctor's assistant.

'The wound is blind,' the doctor's assistant said after looking at the political instructor closely. 'It's bad. If a bullet touches a rib, it often changes direction. Then to find it without an X-ray...'

Suddenly the wounded man opened his eyes slightly. Staring at the face of the battalion doctor's assistant, he rasped, 'You, Maltsev?'

'Yes, it's me, Comrade Political Instructor. A medical instructor and stretcher-bearers are with me. Now we'll send you...'

'Send them first,' the political instructor looked towards the wounded soldiers, lying on the far side of the dugout. 'Things look very bad for them.'

'We'll help everyone, Comrade Political Instructor; we'll get them all out,' Maltsev encouraged Bystrov while bandaging the lieutenant.

'Send them first,' he repeated, staring at the doctor's assistant and gasping for air. 'That's an order!'

'Yes, Comrade Political Instructor!' the sergeant said curtly. 'Finish the bandaging on your own,' he told Tanya, 'and don't forget to give a tetanus injection.'

Remembering something, the doctor's assistant ran out of the dugout. Soon he returned with a thing which looked like a suitcase to Tanya. The doctor's assistant put the suitcase on the earthen floor and gave an order: 'Give tea from the flask to everyone except those with stomach wounds, of course. Take the cup from the kit.'

With these words Maltsev stepped into the darkness of the dugout and kept on examining the wounded. Tanya joined him after she had distributed the hot tea, which smelled of pine needles. Maltsev gave her an inquisitive look, and she answered, 'I did everything, Comrade Sergeant, as you ordered. And I covered him with a greatcoat.'

Nodding, the doctor's assistant untied his torch from the ceiling and shone it towards a wounded soldier, lying on his stomach.

'Roll up his tunic and shirt and pull down his trousers to his knees. But be careful.'

Having examined the wounded soldier, Maltsev frowned and said, 'Spinal column. Shrapnel. He seems unconscious. There is not much blood on the bandage. That means that the shock is algetic. The spinal cord may be injured. Give him two injections – anti-tetanus and an analgetic solution. You'll find them in my kit. I'll call the stretcher-bearers.'

The doctor's assistant came back with two soldiers. 'The bunk is fixed to the poles with wire. Clean it and you'll carry the wounded soldier on it,' Maltsev instructed the stretcher-bearers. Turning to Tanya, he continued: 'Now we shall change the bandage, dress him and tie his legs and arms to the bunk. Immobilization of the spine in such cases is the main thing.'

The wounded soldier was carefully taken out of the dugout. Again, some machine guns began to rattle from the German side. Bullets whistled over the heads of the soldiers, who dropped to the ground, as crimson trails of fire streaked the air.

'You won't get the wounded man back alive if you crawl,' the doctor's assistant said doubtfully to the stretcher bearer, who was lying nearby. If you push him along, the soldier will die. You'll have to carry him in a crouch and be careful.'

'We'll do it, Comrade Sergeant, we have done it before.'

Maltsev nodded, crawled to the entrance of the dugout and dove inside.

'I can't feel his pulse, Comrade Sergeant,' Tanya said to the doctor's assistant with agitation.

'We can't help him,' Maltsev said gloomily and took his hand off the soldier's carotid artery. 'The loss of blood is too great; his tunic is wet through. The soldier won't survive…'

From the opposite corner of the dugout a loud groan was heard – on the earthen floor a thin soldier, white-faced like a sheet of paper, was writhing in pain and holding his stomach with both hands. Maltsev pushed aside the soldier's arms with one movement. Tanya removed the dressing, applied by someone during the fight, and gasped with fright at intestines that had slipped out of the abdominal cavity.

'Shall I tuck them back in?' Tanya exclaimed.

'Not on your life!' Maltsev said sharply. 'Get the bearer quickly, he is at the entrance. And take the canteen.'

Giving the arms of the wounded to the bearer, the doctor's assistant wetted the bandage he had taken from the packet, and put it into the casualty's mouth. The patient pressed his teeth into it, trying to suck the water. Having applied a new dressing, Maltsev said quickly: 'Get the rest for the examination,' and he and the bearer took the soldier out of the dugout.

In five minutes, the doctor's assistant returned smelling of ether. Glancing at the medical instructor, he said in a low voice, 'I put him out fof his misery, as his condition was hopeless. He was in agony.'

'Shall we leave him here?' Tanya asked.

'We'll have to,' the voice of the sergeant sounded like metal. 'Later his body will be carried out by the medical orderlies. And we must evacuate those who have a chance to survive. We have half an hour,' he added gloomily.

'The torch will soon go out, and I couldn't find any spare batteries in the battalion storehouse. We have to double the tempo.'

'This wounded man has no visible injuries. I examined him all over, but he is unconscious,' Tanya looked at the sergeant in surprise.

Maltsev quickly touched the body of the soldier, sounded his lungs, felt his pulse, examined his eyes and made concluded, 'He has a concussion, a severe one, and must be sent to the medical battalion as soon as possible.'

Mishin ran into the dugout. He informed them excitedly, 'Alma is barking. She feels the presence of newcomers nearby. I think German medics are also looking for their wounded. That's why their machine guns are silent.'

'Help me, please!' the sergeant ordered, raising the legs of the concussed soldier. They carried the soldier out in the open.

'Put him on the stretcher, quickly, and leave,' Maltsev whispered to two soldiers who were sitting near a bush. 'The Germans are not far away.'

A tall stretcher bearer held out a grenade with a long wooden handle to the doctor's assistant, 'Take it, Comrade Sergeant, it might be useful. It is the one I took from the German, when we were crawling here.'

Maltsev suddenly remembered that when transporting the political instructor, he caught sight of the barrel of some weapon, hanging on the corner pole of the dugout.

'This is the political instructor's gun!' exclaimed Mishin gladly as he slid his hand along the barrel. 'He always took it into battle…are there any cartridges or is it empty?'

Maltsev shrugged his shoulders. Removing the magazine, the guide weighed it in his palm and confidently concluded, 'It will be enough for two short bursts.'

'Then we live, don't we, Alma?' the guide gave the dog

a pat on the head. Spreading a greatcoat near the shrub, Mishin waved his hand reassuringly. 'If there is something, I'll drive them away. Their medics are only armed with pistols. They have no reason to look for a scrap. I'll keep watch over the entrance to the dugout, and Alma won't let them get close unnoticed from the rear.'

The torch had lost its energy and lit the dugout so weakly that Maltsev at first couldn't find the figure of the medical instructor in the darkness. Tanya was kneeling with a syringe in her hand near the wounded soldier.

'Comrade Sergeant, I gave him an antitetanic injection, and changed the bandage on his head, but the tourniquet on the right leg is applied below the knee.'

'Tourniquet? All this time?!'

The doctor's assistant took a box of matches and lit some of them. The flame brightly lit the wounded soldier.

'Roll up his pant leg, quickly!'

Swearing, Maltsev changed the matches and carefully examined the soldier's leg. Waving his hand slightly, he asked Tanya, 'You changed the dressing. What's the matter with his head?'

'A small wound, the bone is not injured.'

'Not injured, you say, and the soldier is unconscious.'

Thinking, the doctor's assistant rubbed his chin. 'It's perhaps from loss of blood or shock from the pain. The artery behind his knee is damaged. The tourniquet is to be left on the leg not less than a day. The leg will probably be amputated, but his life can be saved. So now, everybody back to your places, and quickly. Two minutes to prepare. I'll go and find out what's going on.'

'How are the fascists?' Maltsev asked Mishin, who was lying in his usual pose.

'Civilized,' the guide joked, 'they are not bothering us.'

'Maybe Alma frightened them?' the doctor's assistant kept up the joke.

The sergeant admired the quick-witted soldier, who was cheerful in any situation. Together with Mishin they took two wounded soldiers, thermoses, and the kit out of the dugout.

'Tanya, give some tea to the political instructor,' Maltsev ordered, 'and to the wounded soldier, if you can. It's very difficult to bring him round... let me do it!'

'The political instructor is calling you, Comrade Sergeant,' Tanya said while taking the cup from the mouth of the wounded soldier.

'Down below, under my bunk. There are two rifles, take them,' the political instructor whispered, eyes closed, to the doctor's assistant, who was bending over him. Speaking was not easy for him. He was breathing heavily, coughing, and on his pale face there were thick beads of sweat. Mishin brought out two rifles from the dugout. Then he crawled up to the soldier, wounded in the leg, and tried to give him tea.

'The soldier isn't coming to,' he pronounced with regret and hid the cup in the kit, 'So let us have a bit of hot tea.'

Passing the teapot around the circle, the doctor's assistant poured out the rest of the contents of the canteens on the ground. While taking two stretcher straps from the kit, he explained to Tanya, 'We don't need extra kilograms. I'll drag the political instructor, and Mishin will drag the soldier. You have to take the rest—canteens, bags, and the kit. Each of us will take one rifle.'

The sergeant took off his greatcoat, spread it on the ground, inserted the strap into the sleeves and tied the end in a knot. Then he did the same with the guide's greatcoat.

'Two transport units are ready for service,' the sergeant intoned with satisfaction.

Having placed the wounded on the greatcoats, Maltsev and Mishin took the free ends of the straps and dragged the jury-rigged "transport units" to the frontline strong points of the first company.

Tanya was walking alongside and observing the wounded soldiers. She tried not to fall behind. Sometimes she stopped to adjust the heavy rifle, which was sliding from her shoulder. From time to time her glance lingered on the stooped, broad-shouldered figure of Maltsev. The doctor's assistant carefully dragged the greatcoat with the wounded man, holding the loop of the strap over his shoulder.

'How did the sergeant become so knowledgeable in medicine?' This unanswerable question without any answer occupied Tanya's head. 'He is only twenty-five, not more. Perhaps…'

The sharp command "Lie down!" threw Tatyana on the ground. The darkness of the night was again seared by fiery bolts. This time they were green and were whistling over their heads. The guide crawled up to Maltsev: 'It's still about 150 metres from here to our trenches. Shall we wait for the firing to end?'

'We mustn't delay. We must get the wounded to the operating table. We keep going,' the doctor's assistant answered resolutely, and began dragging the wounded soldier, pushing off from the ground with the right and the left leg in turn.

Tanya followed the men's example. She also crawled on one side, dragging the kit and the rifle with one hand and replacing the canteens with the other hand. In the light of the tracer fire over the head, she closed her eyes tight, bent her head close to the ground, but kept on moving.

Alma ran up to them from time to time, who were stubbornly crawling to their destination. She sniffed at everyone, came to a conclusion knowable only to the canine kind, and again ran off ahead.

She led the group to the very trench of the platoon strong point, whence Maltsev, Tanya and their companions had set out for the dugout.

'The company commander was summoned to battalion headquarters. He was interested in the political instructor,' the soldier in a shabby greatcoat reported to the sergeant.

'We'll send them both straight to the divisional medical battalion. They can't be given aid at the regiment medical station', the doctor's assistant hurried the soldiers, and helped carry the wounded to a safe place. 'Their condition is bad. And one more thing from the company command: the dead must be evacuated from the battlefield by dawn.'

'I'm one of the company NCOs, I'm a corporal, Smagin is my name. We'll do everything, Comrade Sergeant, you can be sure!'

Behind the low mound stood the battalion ambulance cart, covered with a tent.

'We were waiting for you, Comrade Sergeant. Glad you arrived!' the short cart driver saluted the sergeant.

'Are you here, Rogov?' Maltsev came up close to the soldier.

'Yes, it's me! We have been waiting for about half an hour.'

'And why do you say "we"? You are the only one here.'

'Me and Mashka,' the driver tapped his whip on the crupper of the horse harnessed to the cart.

Once the wounded had been loaded, Maltsev announced to Rogov 'I'll bring them to the division medical battalion myself. The wounded don't have their medical cards, and the medical battalion commander can refuse to accept them. I have good relations with the commander of the receiving and sorting platoon. I'll fill in the cards there. Clear?'

'Yes, it is,' the driver said dejectedly. 'Or perhaps we'll do it together?'

'No,' the doctor's assistant said sharply. 'You'll take the empty canteens and the two rifles. The automatic gun will remain with me. Clear?'

'It's clear, Comrade Sergeant. Mashka will take you right to the place. She has been there many times, I've lost count.'

'And where am I to go?' Tanya asked the doctor's assistant.

'What do you mean, "where"? Get on the cart. You'll see how the wounded feel and you will take care of them and do everything that is necessary. Let me help you to get into the cart. It's inconvenient to jump in a greatcoat.'

Only now Tanya noticed that the doctor's assistant was standing in a tunic.

'And where is your greatcoat?'

'I used it to cover the wounded, they need the warmth more. Let's go. We must hurry. It's about five kilometres from here to the medical battalion.'

The commander of the triage platoon, an army doctor, met the newcomers almost like enemies. Without hearing Maltsev out, he shouted with irritation,

'Open pneumothorax? Necrosis of a limb? But all our patients have something like that. Look how many we have got!'

The wounded were lying in rows alongside the battalion tents. Their bandages were distinctly white in the dim light of the waxing moon. A stooped orderly was walking along the rows with a cup.

'How many are there, poor things!?' Tanya wondered as she wiped tears away.

Her wordless question seemed to be heard by the doctor. Looking to the side he said sullenly, 'There are forty to be operated on without delay, and in total there are about one hundred wounded men. It will be good if we manage to help them by tomorrow night. For sure, some more will arrive later tonight. We sent both ambulances to the regiment medical station.'

With a tired wave of his hand, he ordered Maltsev, 'Go to the reception room and fill in the newcomers' cards.' After a pause he said in a dry voice, 'I'm sending the political instructor to the operation table right now. Someone was calling and asking about him from division headquarters. The soldiers will have to wait their turn.'

Tanya slept on the way back to the battalion's location. Fatigue and nervous tension did their work. She drifted off after falling on the straw mattresses covering the bottom of the cart.

At the headquarters, the battalion commander, executive officer, and a young dark-haired officer with two cubes on his collar were waiting for Maltsev and Tatyana.

The doctor's assistant saluted and began to report about the fulfillment of the task.

'I know, I heard the report,' the commander stopped the sergeant with a gesture. 'You pulled your fifteenth soldier off the battlefield, correct?'

'I don't remember, Comrade Major,' Maltsev shook his head, 'I didn't count.'

'But the battalion executive officer keeps score properly. Political instructor Bystrov is the fifteenth whom you carried out under fire. Lieutenant Kozlov! Get ready to write the text of the report to the regimental commander,' the battalion commander ordered the black-haired lieutenant.

Looking at Maltsev and Tanya in turn, the major began to dictate in a very serious tone: 'For saving fifteen wounded soldiers and officers by evacuating them from the battlefield, in accordance with the order □ 281, August 23, 1941, issued by the Commissar of Defence of the USSR, Comrade I.V. Stalin, I recommend the doctor's assistant of the medical platoon of the 2nd Infantry Battalion, Sergeant Sergey Nikolayevich Maltsev for the decoration "For Military Merit."

The battalion commander finished dictating the text and asked the doctor's assistant in the same serious voice, 'How did Medical Instructor Rusakova perform?'

The sergeant's answer was a laconic, 'Quickly and accurately.'

'Well done, Comrade Rusakova!' Miroshnikov said, looking at Tanya with respect. 'Your baptism of fire has taken place. I'll announce our gratitude tomorrow morning during roll call.'

'Comrade Major, shall we carry out an order for the battalion?' the black-haired lieutenant asked.

'An order, an order, of course, what else? I am not authorized to issue decrees yet. But that's enough for today. It's time to fulfill Order 0320. Is that clear?'

After closing the thick notebook with satisfaction, the black-haired lieutenant began to place some mugs on the stove.

'What do you think about following the order of the Deputy People's Commissar of Defence of the USSR?' the battalion commander asked Tanya, covering his smile with his hand.

'I…,' the girl was embarrassed. 'I think…the order of the commissar…must be fulfilled.'

'Golden words!' Miroshnikov exclaimed. 'Guram, go for it!'

Jangling the keys, Pichkhadze unlocked the massive safe which stood in the corner and took out a jerry can. Having poured vodka into the mugs and pots, he inquisitively glanced at the battalion commander. Miroshnikov raised his mug, 'Today many of our friends, fighting against the enemy, died as brave soldiers, and many of them are wounded. But we threw the Germans back, and they will never win. We're fighting for the Motherland.'

The battalion commander paused and looked at Tatyana. 'Women help us men fight the fascists. And even young women join us. The German "Frau" cannot compare!'4

The major emptied the mug in two gulps and glanced at the girl, 'What are you waiting for? You have had your baptism of fire today and it's not a sin to have a cup of drink. It's an order from the high command.'

'I never drink spirits,' red in the face, Tanya shook her head in despair. 'Never! And it is vodka, I'm sorry!'

She quickly added her portion to the mug of the battalion commander.

'She fulfilled Order 0320, Comrade Major,' Pichkhadze said while opening a tin of food with a knife.

'How is that?' the battalion commander stared at his assistant. 'Explain.'

'I was told about this order at divisional headquarters last year. There was some kind of affair at the end of August. The order was telegraphed.'

---

4   woman (German)

'In August or in September makes no difference. What are you getting at?'

'The order says that a soldier is to be given 100 grams every day, but as to what he is to do with the vodka, there is not a single word.' The flame of the lamp began to dance as if it were trying to flee the dugout.

'You should try to go into acting, Guram, after the war. You'll be taken by any theatre, even without a diploma,' the battalion commander said, after he stopped coughing and wiped his reddened face. He was pleased.

He put the handkerchief in his pocket, and looked at the face of his watch, glowing in the darkness of the tent and announced, 'My brave men, we all need a rest. The fascists are brazen. In the morning they will probably launch an offensive again. Oh, I see that the medical instructor cannot keep her legs under her. And we are no better.'

Putting his hand on the black-haired lieutenant's shoulder, he said:

'I say, Kozlov, the executive officer will manage the orders by himself. And you go quickly to the first company to strengthen it, you'll take command of the first platoon. Senior Lieutenant Zhelnov is the only officer left there.'

Maltsev and Tanya left the dugout. The doctor's assistant said,

'You'll sleep in the warehouse tonight. This is temporary. We medics have our personal dugout, but right now we've got too many wounded men. That's why we decided to put some of them in the dugout. Tomorrow we'll evacuate them and then...'

'Don't worry, please' Tanya waved her hands. 'I'll spend the night wherever you say.'

'Good. In the warehouse there are some sacks and parcels with underwear, they'll make a soft bed. And the rats won't bother you. They are frightened by the smell of medicine.'

In the warehouse, a mud hut with a roof barely seen above the ground, the doctor's assistant lit some matches and put the padlock on the shelf. 'On the door there is a latch; lock it from inside,' he said, waving good-bye.

'And where will he sleep at night, if the wounded soldiers lie in the dugout?' Tanya thought in distress, but soon she was deep asleep. Her dreams swept her thoughts and feelings away.

In the morning Miroshnikov called her in. Chewing a match, the battalion commander silently pointed at a box covered with a piece of material. When Tanya sat down on the edge of the makeshift stool, he began talking slowly, choosing his words. 'Once, in the first company there was a nurse who worked as a medical instructor. She was as young as you are; well, perhaps a little older.'

'She was twenty-two, Comrade Major,' Pichkhadze chimed in and stopped playing with the telephone receiver.

'It's not important,' the battalion commander waved his hand. 'The important thing was that she received many soldiers at night. Do you get it?'

'No, no.' Tanya shook her head.

'I'll explain' Miroshnikov said in a dry voice. 'There are a hundred and fifty boys and young men in the company. So she received them one after the other after taps,[5] nearly

---

5   Bugle call at dusk.

ten a night. In the end the company commander and the
political instructor found out about it and stopped such
disgraceful behaviour.'

'Why are you telling me this, Comrade Major,?' Tanya
exclaimed with indignation. 'I won't give them a chance—'

The battalion commander waved his hand to in
recognition,

'You won't give a chance to anyone, I see that. But
people are different, aren't they? And you are such an
attractive girl. For example, a few wayward men will likely
conspire to rape you; they might rush into the tent and
you won't be able to utter a sound or raise hell. That is
why you should follow my orders. You may only be with
the company in the daytime, more precisely, from reveille
to taps. After that—'

Miroshnikov failed to finish his sentence. Three
explosions thundered quite close to the dugout, one after
another.

'Here they come, the devils!' the battalion commander
cursed and began to quickly turn over the mugs and
kettles on the barrel.

'They are firing their 80-milimetre guns,' Pichkhadze
said gloomily and began to hide magazines and papers in
the safe. Miroshnikov spun the handle of the telephone
and shouted into the receiver,

'Connect me with the 10th, quickly!'

He tried to calm down Tanya, who had turned pale,
and said 'The fascists can't get us with their shells – the
dugout roof has three layers made of thick logs, and all
that is covered with half a metre of soil. It will withstand

even a direct hit. But earth and sand pour through the ceiling and spoil the documents.'

On receiving a report from an unknown man over the telephone, the battalion commander cheered up, saying, 'It's calm at the front line. Obviously, the Germans targeted the headquarters. They haven't forgotten us. Yesterday, and three days ago, they sent us the same presents.'

'The day before yesterday the observation post reported that a 'rama'6 was circling above. Would it be better to move the headquarters to an alternate position?' Pichkhadze took a folded map out of the bag and came up to Miroshnikov. 'Maybe here, at the copse.'

'We'll have to change the observation system and build new dugouts and shelters. It's a bit of a problem, but it seems we'll have to,' the battalion commander agreed unwillingly. 'Life is more important.'

Maltsev entered the dugout in a hurry.

'Shells are thudding around, and he is running as if it were a sports competition!' Miroshnikov all but attacked the doctor's assistant. 'What's up? Fire? Flood?'

'Seems so, Comrade Major, they have typhus in the first company. There are two patients.'

'What did you say?!' the battalion commander roared so fiercely that both Pichkhadze and Tatyana jumped up and froze.

---

6   *A German reconnaissance plane, the Focke Wulf 189.*

***

'If it's not Germans, it's typhus! Poor things!' Miroshnikov began to swear at the enemy, but soon he pulled himself together. 'Report, Sergeant, what you've done about it and what is still to be done.'

'Both patients are isolated. The medical orderlies are preparing a cart. We'll take the patients straight to the medical battalion. We'll put fir branches in the cart, and we'll disinfect the mattresses. We have to examine the whole company. Then we must organize the bathing of the entire company. Then we'll disinfect the underwear, uniforms, and footwear.'

'Your plan, Sedoy, is perfect,' Miroshnikov encouraged him. 'However, where can I get ahold of a bath-house, spare uniforms, and bedding – for one hundred men?'

'We'll pitch a tent near the bog and camouflage it. Then we'll dig a hole and put a barrel with water on a fire. That'll do for hot water, and we can put another barrel for cold water in the tent. We'll disinfect the boots and uniforms over the fire.'

'Alright, Sedoy, get to work!' the battalion commander decisively sliced the air with his hand. 'I promise to provide uniforms for changing. The medical instructor will help you. And you, clearly, head off to the company straight away. Rusakova will catch up with you.'

'Yes, Sir!', the doctor's assistant saluted and quickly left the dugout.

'How do you like Maltsev?' the commander asked Tatyana, with half-closed eyes.

Tatyana felt she was blushing. But suddenly she burst out, 'Well, he is... he is a real talent! So much knowledge, so much experience, I can't imagine where from...'

The major stopped the girl's excited speech with a gesture, 'From where? He graduated from the Leningrad medical institute with honors. He refused a post-graduate education at the institute. He asked to be sent to the district hospital, because he wanted to gain experience first. Three years later he became head physician there.'

Miroshnikov sighed and stopped talking. Looking gloomily at the cast-iron door of the stove, he drummed his fingers on the bottom of the kettle.

'And then?' Tatyana was struck by the news.

Tanya felt that she shouldn't have asked the battalion commander this question.

'Then there were changes in his life. That'll do,' Miroshnikov said in a cold voice. 'Catch up with the sergeant. Drop by at the supply platoon and tell the commander to come here.'

Though Tanya hurried to reach the first company to help Maltsev in sending the typhus patients to the hospital battalion, she was too late. The doctor's assistant and the company commander were sitting on the thick trunk of a fallen tree. They were discussing the examination and disinfection of the soldiers. The medical cart, familiar to Tatyana, was raising dust along the dirt road which led into the depths of the forest. It was driven by Rogov and the mare, Mashka.

'Why are you, Comrade Medical Instructor, marching around at full height? You are not on main street!' the company commander remarked to Tanya. 'The Germans have good snipers. At the front line there are three possible ways of moving – on your stomach, on all fours, and crouching, is that clear?'

'Clear, Comrade Captain!' Tanya uttered distinctly.

'And if it is clear, then hurry with the doctor's assistant to the bog using one of those methods. I'll send company soldiers there.'

Near a small pond (measuring about fifteen by twenty steps), with a grassy shore and full of pond scum, about ten soldiers and the commander of the supply platoon were pottering about. Two of them were fashioning stakes for a tent, and the others were digging a hole for water barrels.

Maltsev chose a place to pitch the tent and came up to the commander of the platoon, a short first sergeant in a short, faded uniform. 'Not far away, behind the shrubs, a small gully begins, we'll put up a tent there,' he told the man.

'Why? Are you crazy?' the sergeant shouted in Ukrainian. 'We'll have fifty or more steps to carry the hot water!'

'We'll have to dig a pit in the gully,' the doctor's assistant continued quietly. 'That way the snipers won't notice the tent.'

'That's right, Comrade Sergeant,' the executive officer said, as he and the medical platoon commander approached the bog.

'Show me and Petrenko the sanitary inspection station location,' Pichkhadze ordered.

Cursing under their breath, the soldiers of the supply

platoon left the half-dug pit with regret. On checking the approaches to the ravine, the executive officer nodded with satisfaction, 'That's good! There is a slope. Water will run away from the tent.' Then, looking at his watch, he announced, 'Get ready to examine the soldiers of the first company at twelve sharp. Seventy sets of new uniforms will be delivered from the regiment. They promised. Find thirty more. That is your task, Comrade Petrenko.'

'Thirty!?' Petrenko said with dismay. 'Where will I find them?'

'Wherever you want, just get them!' the executive officer said angrily. 'You can even undress your diggers, but soldiers at the front line must be in properly uniformed and shod. By the way, how many soldiers of the company have long boots?'

'About fifty. The rest are in puttees.'

'I know that they aren't in dress shoes. Autumn is coming, and those in the rear are loafing. This concerns you as well, Comrade First Sergeant.'

'But two weeks ago I sent a request for three hundred pairs. For all the companies…'

'Two weeks ago! You must send requests every day! Send them another one today, by special delivery.' Snapping his fingers, Pichkhadze turned to Maltsev:

'What are you going to do with the footwear of the soldiers?'

'Body lice can be found in clothing seams, head lice are found in the hair. But they can also get into boots. That's why we'll disinfect the footwear by holding them over the fire. The lice don't like the heat and die quickly at 80 degrees Centigrade.'

'All right, Sergeant. Get started. If you need me, I'll be in the headquarters.' Hunching over, Pichkhadze headed for the battalion.

The platoon commander, a stooping, middle-aged, ruddy-faced junior lieutenant, came up to Maltsev. As if apologizing he said, 'I can't help you, Sedoy, there are many wounded soldiers in the battalion, we're out of space. During the night orderlies and stretcher-bearers brought in twenty-six more. You and the medical instructor will have to deal with the infectious cases.

'Of course, no problem!' Maltsev waved his hand encouragingly. 'We'll manage, Viktor Ivanovich.'

The medical platoon commander nodded and hurried after Pichkhadze.

The supply platoon commander informed the doctor's assistant he would be off to find the uniforms and also left.

Two soldiers appeared in the ravine, carrying stakes. Tanya made an effort to help with the tent, but Maltsev objected: 'Your time will soon come, and we three men, will manage it ourselves.'

Waiting for the doctor's assistant and the soldiers to finish putting up the tent, Tanya approached the pit, where eight soldiers were shoveling clayish soil onto the slopes of the ravine.

'Smoke break, boys!' a lanky soldier wiped the sweat from his forehead and joyfully glanced at the girl. 'Time for a physical. Keep away. I'm the first to be examined!'

'How do you like that, Vanya is the first!' a black-eyed

robust fellow, covered in clay, objected. 'As soon as the medical instructor looks at your bones, she'll faint. But I have something to show.'

The soldier winked at Tanya and deftly jumped out of the pit. Then he pronounced in a sugary voice, 'What's your name then, Comrade Medical Instructor?

Tanya didn't answer. When the black-eyed boy jumped out of the pit, she noticed a red spot on his neck. She gave a strict order: 'Turn around, quickly!'

'From behind?' the heavy-set young man threw up his hands with a smile. 'I've never been with a woman that way.'

Soon Tanya was behind him and quickly straightened out the collar of his tunic. On his neck, she saw a big red boil.

'Does it ache?' Tanya touched the red spot with her fingers. It was hot to the touch.

'Not much, it will go away soon,' the soldier turned to Tanya and began to look at her slender figure with admiration.

'Well, what's your name?'

'Let's go!' Tatyana said, and marched him to the medical assistant.

The large, partially-pitched tent was flapping in the wind. Maltsev and two soldiers were trying vainly to stretch the uncooperative canvas onto the stakes.

'Grab the free corner!' the sergeant ordered Tanya and her patient.

***

Soon the tent was pitched properly, divided into two sections. Maltsev examined the structure critically and paced off the distance from the entrance to the opposite wall.

'It's alright!' the doctor's assistant turned to Tanya, pleasure on his face. 'What's the matter with the soldier?'

'A problem with his neck,' Tanya turned back the greasy collar of the soldier's tunic.

'A carbuncle,' Maltsev diagnosed, looking at the boil. 'It must be lanced and drained urgently.'

'Comrade Sergeant,' the young man pleaded, hands pressed to his breast, 'Don't you cut it, I had something similar on my leg, but now everything is quite all right. I can't stand iodine and medicine…'

'First of all, Comrade Soldier, stay still,' Maltsev interrupted him sharply. 'A leg isn't a neck. From there, the infection can get into your brain. Then you're done for.'

The doctor's assistant's last words frightened the soldier. Noticing, Maltsev said softly, 'I hope that won't happen. We'll finish the medical treatment, and I'll do what you need.' Looking at Tanya, he shrugged his shoulders.

'It's striking! The soldier isn't afraid of German bullets, but he nearly loses consciousness from the smell of iodine.'

The supply platoon commander entered the tent. Soldiers with carrying packages followed him. Breathing heavily after a quick walk, the first sergeant said, 'Twenty-three uniforms. I have taken the whole battalion's supply. But I only found three pairs of wearable boots. Ten pieces of soap: they must be spent carefully. There are a lot of towels: last month we made them from old sheets. There are two packages of underwear. I think it will be enough for everyone. And I found a washtub. There are only two basins, and one has no handles. But there are nine pails!'

The first sergeant pushed his field cap upwards, scratched his forehead and said thoughtfully, 'It makes no difference where you splash – in a basin or in a pail. I'll walk to the pit and see what my boys have done.'

In the earthen dugout, a metre and a half deep, the soldiers of the supply platoon, under the guidance of the first sergeant Petrenko, had made two fires. Over one of them they put a two-hundred-litre barrel, with the help of stones from the bog. The dry branches were rapidly crackling in the fire, and the water in the barrel was soon warm. Over the second fire, the soldiers hung some poles for disinfecting underwear.

They put another two barrels in the main part of the tent. One was filled with cold water and the second they planned for hot water from the pit. Cut into logs, the thick trunk of the fallen tree was used by the doctor's assistant and the medical instructor as a table and stools.

Maltsev sent the black-eyed soldier to the forest to cut spruce branches and spread them on the floor of the smaller part of the tent.

'The water will soon begin to boil,' the commander of the supply platoon said as he appeared in the tent, snapping his pocket watch shut. 'It's midday already. They have fallen asleep in the company, haven't they?'

'They'll come,' Maltsev waved his hand to calm everyone down. 'And where's Sinitsyn, our barber?'

'He was to have come long ago,' the first sergeant said in frustration. 'Oh, that devil! He'll get three days' extra duty,' the sergeant continued in Ukrainian.

He didn't have to impose the penalty: Sinitsyn, a fair-haired soldier in puttees, with a thin kit-bag in his hand, slipped into the tent. He was followed by a black-haired soldier, who reported that the floor had been covered with spruce branches.

'Fair words fill not the belly. I'd rather deal with you!' Maltsev said, looking at him.

'What's your surname?'

'Gambarov, Comrade Sergeant.'

'And your first name?'

'Rustam. Maybe now's not a good time, Comrade Sergeant?'

'Stop talking!' the doctor's assistant frowned, turned the soldier so he could see his back and examined the carbuncle.

Thinking for a second, he ordered: 'Get undressed. You may have another one in some other place.'

Rustam took off his boots, tunic and trousers and cast a sidelong look at the girl who was sitting on a log. Noticing that the soldier was uncomfortable, Tanya turned around and began to take everything out of the first aid kit on the nearby stool.

'Medical Instructor Rusakova,' the voice of the doctor's assistant sounded unusually cold. 'Take part in the examination. Very soon the soldiers of the first company will be streaming in. I won't manage alone.'

Blushing to the roots of her hair, Tanya jumped up and ran to the sergeant.

'I won't undress if there's a woman here!' Gamburov said and shook his head at Tanya. 'Send her away!'

Platoon Commander Petrenko jumped into the conversation. 'Private Gamburov!' the first sergeant's eyes narrowed. 'You will obey all orders given by the doctor's assistant and the medical instructor! Otherwise you'll answer to me...!'

Glancing at the melon-sized fists of the platoon commander, Gamburov sighed and began to take off his shirt. Standing half-naked, he remarked resentfully, 'Will you measure anything?'

Maltsev looked at his groin and parried, 'We don't have a micrometer at our disposal.'

Tanya stopped herself from bursting out laughing.

'What don't you have?' Gamburov hadn't caught the word.

'Nothing,' Petrenko, who was standing nearby, hissed, 'You've been told to keep quiet, so keep quiet.'

'There are no more infiltrates,' the doctor's assistant said after examining the body of the soldier.

'Hey, wait!' Maltsev squatted. 'What have we got here?'

On Gambarov's scrotum there were several small, dark cherry-coloured knots. The doctor's assistant touched them lightly with his hand.

'Spread your fingers apart!' he ordered the soldier, who frightfully followed the actions of the sergeant.

'Pay attention,' Maltsev invited Tatyana to look at the wrinkles between the fingers. 'These small grayish stripes that look like scratches, are mite tracks. The eruption in the groin is secondary – the infected soldier brought mites there with his hands. I'm sure, on the penis it'll be the same story. Examine, please.' Tanya shook her head in despair.

'Well, well,', Maltsev said mildly, seeing the state of the girl. 'I'll explore it myself. But remember, you'll have to examine all the soldiers in the company every month this way.'

The doctor's assistant bared the head of the penis with a quick movement and diagnosed the disease.

'Scabies!' Looking at the pale face of Gamburov, he comforted the soldier, 'Nothing dangerous, Rustam. We'll treat you: actually, you'll do it yourself under my observation.'

'Nothing bad!?' Petrenko's face grew red with indignation. 'He'll infect the whole platoon! Send him to the medical battalion right away!

'Scabies will take at least month of treatment,' Maltsev objected, trying to speak in a quiet tone. 'There are not enough specialists to save people's lives in the medical battalion. Scabies should be treated here.'

Two soldiers from the supply platoon entered the tent with pails of hot water.

'Pour it into the last barrel!' the doctor's assistant ordered. 'And one more thing,' Maltsev turned to Petrenko, 'we must send Maslovsky someone. I'll write him a message.'

'No problem. Hey, Yerokhin, wait a little!' the first sergeant stopped one of the soldiers, who was on his way out. 'Take this message to the commander of the medical platoon, Comrade Maslovsky.

'Why are you standing like a pylon!?' Petrenko shouted at Gamburov. 'The hot water is here. Take the basin. You don't remember when you washed your neck the last time, do you?'

'Not yet,' Maltsev stopped the first sergeant. 'First we must administer a hyposulphite sodium and muriatic acid solution. He will do it every day. Then five days later he'll wash himself.'

From outside, tramping feet and muted laughter were heard. The front section of the tent was filled with soldiers of the first company, who had arrived for examination.

'Quiet! Don't chatter!' the commander of the supply platoon admonished. 'Take it all off, including your knickers. You'll get one piece of soap for two men, and a pair of underwear after washing; then you each get a change of uniform once you sign this paper.'

When ten stark naked soldiers entered the main part of the tent, Tanya felt herself break into a sweat. She had seen a naked man only once in her life, when she studied to be a nurse. The courses were organized at the hospital, where she had been sent by the military committee after graduating from the medical school's obstetrics department. That patient was a wounded middle-aged soldier; the wound was in the lower part of the stomach. Tatyana had changed the bandage under the watchful eye of the senior nurse.

The doctor's assistant saw the girl's embarrassment. He came up close to Tanya and said quietly, 'We are physicians, they are just patients. We'll start simultaneously and work fast. As far as the rash is concerned, you saw it. Don't miss typhus rash. Spotted fever has an incubatory period of two weeks and even more. It's difficult to identify every case.'

'Where's our barber?' Maltsev called to Sinitsyn, who was standing bored in the corner, with a gesture. 'Everyone gets a shave: close-cropped head, armpits and groin a complete shave.'

After having their hair cut and being examined, the soldiers took the basins and pails, and washed each other.

'Here is Yerokhin!' the first lieutenant exclaimed, pleased to see the soldier in the tent. 'You are very quick, good show.'

'I ran there and back, Comrade First Lieutenant,' the soldier said with a satisfied grin, and held out his package.

'Give it to the doctor's assistant,' Petrenko ordered.

Maltsev fussed over the package for a while, before stirring the contents into a pail of hot water. Then he instructed Gamburov, who was sitting in the tent corner wrapped in a greatcoat, 'Wet the towel in this liquid and rub it into your body, especially your hands and feet, groin, and armpits. Rub it into your head, too. Do it in the corner. But first go to Sinitsyn for a haircut.'

They heard voices outside.

'It looks like someone has arrived from the company,' the first lieutenant said, and dove energetically into the other room. Just as quickly he was back, rubbing his hands with pleasure. 'That's right – no less than thirty uniforms and pairs of boots.' Picking up a dirty notebook from one of the stools, he popped out again.

After the soldiers were disinfected and had changed their underwear, they left the tent for the company. Petrenko glanced at his watch and said gloomily,

'Midday is right around the corner. You cut your hair and washed yourselves for more than an hour. Heaven forbid we finish after dark. And I am to organize dinner for the companies.'

'How are things, Rustam? Have you rubbed your hands and feet well?' Maltsev came up to Gambarov. 'Let me rub your back. No…the medical instructor will do it. And I'll go check on the uniform and boot disinfection.'

The doctor's assistant did not manage to do what he had planned. A runner from headquarters came in. After saluting, he held out a message to the sergeant. Maltsev read it and swore. He glanced at Tatyana in confusion and said, 'The battalion commander orders you to come immediately. Some authorities have come from divisional headquarters. They are interested in you.'

'Me?' Tanya was astonished. 'But I've only been at the front for one day.'

'I don't understand it either,' Maltsev murmured. 'Though, probably…'

'Well, I never! What will you do here alone? I must… my goodness! It's high time to feed the men too! It's my most important duty!' Petrenko cursed the brass and HQ. 'Well, Sedoy, be a man! I'll send the platoon commander, Sergeant Gusev. He's bright, he will help you.'

'There's nothing for it, Tanya. You have to go,' the

doctor's assistant nodded to the girl encouragingly. 'But drop in at the medical station and tell Maslovsky about the situation.'

After putting everything she had taken out earlier back into the bag, Tanya headed for the exit. Before stepping out she looked back, caught the assistant's glance, and smiled faintly.

In the headquarters dugout sat two unfamiliar officers, the battalion commander, and the executive officer. Tanya saw one rectangle on the blue collar of one of them. The second man was sitting on one of the bunks in such a position that Tanya couldn't make out his rank. The young woman saluted and began to report to the battalion commander.

'Take a seat, Comrade Rusakova,' interrupted the officer with blue lapel tabs, and pointed at the familiar canvas-covered box. After a few minutes of silence, he began to ask questions.

'Last night you participated in the treatment and evacuation of wounded in a dugout in No Man's Land. Your group was led by the doctor's assistant, Sergeant Maltsev. What can you say about his actions in fulfilling the mission?'

'Perhaps he'll receive a higher decoration, maybe that's why they want more details,' Tatyana thought to herself and answered confidently, 'He was brave and exemplary. He diagnosed the wounds quickly, with confidence and precision... I've never seen anything like it...'

'Well, you haven't seen much,' the officer interrupted her again. He looked at Tatyana coldly.

'We know that the doctor's assistant didn't want to help the company political instructor, Senior Lieutenant Bystrov,' the officer, who had come out of the shadows, said. 'Moreover, he didn't evacuate the badly wounded officer immediately. He should have done that first and foremost.'

Only then did Tanya see the crimson rectangles on his tunic lapel.

'No, no! The sergeant did nothing of the sort,' she objected, looking wide-eyed at the officers. 'The sergeant diagnosed a pneumothorax right away and bandaged the political instructor. And he didn't evacuate him because the instructor himself gave the order not to.'

'What order? Can you clarify?' the officer snapped, scrutinizing Tatyana from under the thick black brows that met at the bridge of his nose.

'The political instructor ordered him to help the soldiers first.'

'Did he really?'

'Yes, he did!' Tanya said firmly. 'The doctor's assistant wanted to evacuate him after dressing his wound, but the instructor said, "First evacuate the Red Army soldiers. I order you!"'

'So that's how it went,' the officer responded. His eyes, watching the expression on the girl's face, were getting warmer.

'Who else can confirm the political instructor's words? Was there anyone else in the dugout at that moment besides you and the doctor's assistant?' asked the officer with blue tabs.

'Only us and the wounded,' Tanya answered. 'The guide and the stretcher-bearers stayed at the entrance. The political instructor can confirm that himself, can't he?'

'Possibly, if he regains consciousness,' said the officer in a cold biting tone.

'So he, as it turns out, was not only a hero in battle, he also saved those privates at the cost of his own life,' the officer with red buttonholes thought and shrugged his shoulders. Addressing Miroshnikov, he declared, 'We'll decorate Bystrov. What decoration? We'll think it over at the division headquarters and then decide. And we'll publish an article in the army newspaper, or maybe send material to the central newspaper, to Comrade Vadimov. I'll telephone you later today, Commander. You'll write a recommendation. And now let's go to your positions. The executive officer will join us. I haven't been here for a long time.'

The officers, excepting the one with blue tabs, ducked their heads and went out.

'You, Comrade Rusakova, showed your worth in fulfilling the mission,' he said as he fixed his eyes on Tanya. 'My name is Kucherenko. I read your personal dossier, as I'm with the special department of the division. You are a Komsomol member, and you are well thought of. I think you can help in the struggle against fascism, and not only as a medic.'

'What other way is there?' she blurted out in astonishment.

'This is how,' the man continued in a patronizing tone. 'Every citizen of our country, especially a Red Army soldier, must be vigilant. And in time of war, doubly so. Fourteen months into the struggle, we must face the facts. We have cowards, alarmists, and traitors in our ranks – there are even enemy spies among us. Exposing them is quite difficult, you see. I am making myself clear?'

'But I…I can't expose them, we were not taught to do that,' Tanya exclaimed. She didn't understand what the officer meant.

'Not everybody is taught to expose enemies, but everybody should be watchful. You know the proverb "Like father, like son," don't you? Is it true?'

'I think it is.' Tanya shrugged her shoulders.

'Absolutely true, like all folk wisdom. And now listen. Sergeant

Maltsev is the son of an enemy,' lowering his voice, Kucherenko pronounced each word deliberately, quietly, watching Tanya's reaction. Embarrassed by his words, Tatyana lowered her eyes. Her hands began to pull at the hem of her tunic.

'Let's suppose,' the officer of the special department continued, looking up at the dugout's log ceiling, 'Sergeant Maltsev, unlike his father, is going to serve the Motherland with devotion. Such things do happen among relatives. But citizens with such "spots" in their biographies must always be under observation,' Kucherenko raised his index finger, 'Constant observation of the special departments and their assistants. And you, Rusakova, will help us in this case.' The officer stopped talking and waited for the girl to react.

Tanya was silent. Her mind raced chaotically — she couldn't think straight in this situation. But she understood one thing: the officer's suspicion was groundless.

'What does "going to serve honestly" mean?' she thought, the officer's words grating on her ears. 'Doesn't he understand that Maltsev is fighting against enemies right now, selflessly risking his life, and they doubt him.'

'I've only known the sergeant for one day, but I learned a lot about him.' Tanya insisted as she pulled herself together. 'He, I'm sure, is devoted to the cause. He makes sure...'

'Only one day, you say?' the officer smiled. 'What does folk wisdom say? To learn what a person is, one must eat a pud of salt with him. This doesn't only apply to Maltsev. In your company, we need vigilant eyes and ears. What is the soldiers' morale? What do they speak about? I need comprehensive data.'

Having thought a little, Kucherenko stood up from the bed. Tanya also jumped up from the stool.

'In a week or two you'll be called to the regimental medical station. I'll arrange it,' the officer said coldly. 'You'll get my instructions there. Not a word to anyone about our conversation. Dismissed.'

Tatyana's path from battalion headquarters to the first company's medical exam station seemed to be shrouded in fog. To spy, to inform — even for the greater good — was beyond her. Especially as Maltsev had earned her admiration.

A sudden flash passed like lighting through her mind, 'I'll do anything. I'm ready to fulfill any mission, but don't rope me into this business! That's what I'll say to the special department captain.' Tatyana repeated these words aloud again and again, when she thought of her upcoming meeting with Kucherenko at the regiment medical station.

'To whom are you talking?' asked a familiar raspy voice, bringing Tanya out from the multitude of overflowing thoughts.

Near the entrance of the tent, the commander of the supply platoon was sitting on a stump. He was holding a mess tin and eating something greedily. Perhaps it was tasty. 'I'll bring some for you, too.'

Petrenko quickly stood up from the stump and walked towards the ravine. In the corner of the empty tent, Maltsev was bandaging Gamburov's neck.

'The company's having dinner. Food has been brought to us as well. It's barley with a taste of meat,' the doctor's assistant straightened his back. 'And you, Rustam, did very well,' he said with approval. 'In two days come back to be examined. And now go have dinner.'

Gamburov left.

'Did you have dinner yourself?' Tatyana was interested. The doctor's assistant didn't manage to answer, as Petrenko appeared in the tent with two kettles. He put them on the table.

'You are welcome to all we have.' The first sergeant took an aluminum spoon from his belt and gave it to Tatyana. 'The battalion commander allowed me to add stewed meat to the porridge — five tins from the emergency rations. For a hundred men it's a drop in the ocean, but it gives a tasty smell.'

Taking a spoon, Maltsev began to eat. Petrenko ran to fetch the kettle he had left on the stump and joined Tanya and the doctor's assistant. The first sergeant carefully picked the remaining porridge from the bottom, shook his head grievously, and cursed all "Luftwaffe" pilots, without exception.7

'We haven't had bread for three days! The fools have bombed the division bakery. We ate only crusts the first day, and yesterday and today we had short rations. Maybe the supply platoon will manage to bring something before nightfall!'

'Thirty men have been treated,' Maltsev brought Tanya up to speed. 'One with typhus has a fever. He is in the ravine. The medical battalion ambulance is going around the regimental medical stations and should pick him up later. If not, then I'll take him to the medical battalion on horseback in the evening.

'What?' Tanya stopped eating.

'I'll strap him down, and we'll get there slowly.'

'Won't you catch it? He has lice in his clothes and footwear.'

'His clothes and footwear were changed. Typhus isn't an airborne illness. But if a louse bites you, the main thing is not to scratch. Rickettsia is in its excrement, but not in its jaws. If the bite is scratched the skin is damaged, and bacilli get into the body.'

Tanya began to wash the kettles and spoons in hot water.

'The dinner break's too long,' the first sergeant grumbled, looking at his watch.

---

7   German Air Force

'It looks like the next group is approaching,' Maltsev said upon hearing voices outside.

In two minutes, the tent was filled with the next group of soldiers, and the conveyor belt system of examining and treating began again. The supply platoon commander urged the soldiers on, carried water, and gave them clean underwear and uniforms to the soldiers. From time to time he ran to the ravine to check on the disinfection of the next group.

'We can finish it before supper,' the first sergeant said with pleasure,

looking at the nimble hands of the doctor's assistant and the medical instructor.

Suddenly the air was filled with a growing howl, and an instant later a blast shook the tightened canvas of the tent.

'Mortars! Everybody to the ravine, move it!' Petrenko shouted with all his strength.

The soapy soldiers ran out of the tent and rushed to the safety of the ravine. Tanya, Maltsev, and the first sergeant followed them. Somewhere nearby a new blast was heard, then two more. Tree bark rained down on the sheltering soldiers. The doctor's assistant covered the girl with his body.

'The fascists have discovered our little sauna! The bastards! They'll make holes in the barrels and tear the tent to pieces,' pressing himself to the wet ground, Petrenko angrily swore at the German mortarmen in Ukrainian.

The firing stopped as suddenly as it had begun. Now, the artillery boomed and there were a number of bursts somewhere far away from the front line. The first sergeant raised his head and observed, 'Aha! Our gunners have driven the Germans into a corner!'

Listening to the air, he ordered the soldiers, who were lying, still naked, on the grassy slopes of the ravine, 'Look alive, you bums! Into the tent!'

'Skvortsov's been killed, Comrade First Sergeant!'

One of the soldiers lay motionless on his stomach, with his face down on the ground. Maltsev jumped up and ran to his side.

'He's alive,' the doctor's assistant said after he felt pulse on the carotid artery of the wounded soldier. 'It's a splinter wound to the head, and a shoulder wound too..'

The wounded Skvortsov was carried to the tent.

'The canvas roof is torn to shreds,' Petrenko said gloomily, when he saw numerous holes in the top of the tent. 'We'll mend it, of course. And one splinter got the barrel.'

Hot water was streaming from the hole until the first sergeant plugged it with his thumb. He beckoned Sinitsyn and called out, 'Cover this hole with your palm, and I'll make a stopper from some scrap wood. We'll plug the hole, and we're done.'

As he moved away, he ordered the soldiers, 'Don't stay here for long! Wash and dress yourselves and run back to the company.'

Kneeling in the corner, Maltsev bandaged the head of the wounded soldier. The patient groaned and grimaced. Tanya crouched down next to them and began to help the doctor's assistant in silence.

'You'll live, Skvortsov, and even sing,' Maltsev winked at the soldier and finished up the bandaging. 'But you'll have to endure the pain a little while.' Then he explained to Tatyana, 'The fragment left a souvenir gouge in the cranium, and tore off a piece of scalp. It's clear that this is a minor concussion which will heal soon. But the shrapnel ball in the shoulder didn't do much harm – it looks like a ricochet from a tree or a boulder. The blood's just seeping out – major vessels are not affected. It means that the foreign body did not penetrate far, so we can take it out. Give him an antitetanic injection and prepare the area for surgery. I'll go disinfect the instruments in the fire.'

Tanya gave the injection and carefully washed the skin around the wound with soap. Then she rubbed it with iodine.

'That's good!' the doctor's assistant praised Tatyana on his return. He put the instrument box on the stool and rummaged in the medical bag. Then he poured some liquid from the flask onto a piece of cotton. The tent was at once filled with the smell of petrol. Maltsev also wiped the affected area with a tampon.

'Will you pour some water on my hands?' he asked Tanya. 'Oh, and I nearly forgot: give him 70 ml of vodka. The bottle is in my bag.'

The incision revealed the foreign body. It was a ball bearing. Maltsev fidgeted with it and shook his head, 'Those Germans use almost everything. They don't even throw away rusty nails. They fill mortar shells with old ball bearings. This piece of metal hit him on a ricochet, that's why it only penetrated three centimetres.'

Having removed some blood clots, the doctor's assistant stood upand said to Tanya, 'Sprinkle the wound with streptocide and bandage it.'

'And the sutures?'

These wounds don't get stitched. Besides, we haven't got any suturing thread.'

Suddenly Maltsev burst out laughing, 'Skvortsov was lucky. "Every cloud has a silver lining" as the old saying goes, right?'

'What makes you say that?' Tanya glanced at the doctor's assistant in surprise.

'The thing is, he was naked when he was hit. Usually, a bullet or a shell fragment tear through the uniform and pull particles of fabric or dirt into the wound. Complications occur frequently, sometimes even tissue necrosis around the wound.'

Tanya also began laughing and remarked, 'To be naked or as poor as a church mouse isn't always bad, is it?'

The commander of the first company ran into the tent, out of breath.

'I see you lot are happy today,' the senior lieutenant said as he sat down on a log and began to take off his boots. 'I could stand a bath too. I don't remember the last time I had one…what's so funny around here?'

'Because someone was naked,' Maltsev smiled.

'How should I understand that?' the officer stopped taking off his boot and glanced at the medical instructor in confusion. Tanya blushed.

'No, it was Skvortsov, Comrade Senior Lieutenant,' Maltsev explained and pointed at the corner of the tent.

'He was saving himself from the mortars in a negligee.'

'We haven't had anything like that so far!' the company commander laughed and forgot about his boot. 'The men told me everything about the mortar bombardment. Well, if a man wants to live, he'll run to the shelter in his birthday suit if he has to.'

Having removed his boots, the company commander glanced at Tanya and said calmly, 'I've only got a quarter of an hour. Only two officers are left in the company, Kozlov and I. Kozlov got to our location five minutes ago. We must wash quickly.'

'Tanya, go to the fire and tell them to bring hot water.' Maltsev looked into the barrel. 'Six pails.'

The work in the ravine was in full swing. The soldiers of the supply platoon were watching the boots suspended over the fire and flipped them over periodically with sticks.

'No insect can stand this heat!' Petrenko said with a pleased smile. 'What are you looking at, Dzakoyev!?' he suddenly shouted at the thin soldier with a soot-blackened face. 'You're not roasting a chicken! That last boot is smoking. Turn it over, quick!'

Having passed along the order, Tanya returned to the tent, but she dared not enter.

'The men are washing themselves. A wash would do me good too,' Tatyana thought.

She was eager to wash away the sweat, dust, bark, and pine needles that had gotten under her tunic during the shelling, and now itched hotly.

Smoothing down his short hair with his hand, the

commander of the first company came out of the tent, red-cheeked, and smiled good-naturedly, 'My soldiers are digging the dugout. They are working like moles. By evening they'll have finished it. You're welcome to join the company! You are to stay at our location at all times when on duty.'

'The battalion commander ordered me to stay here for a night...'

'I know! You ought to follow orders. I won't insist, but I ensure you that in my company no one will hurt you. You'll be like a sister to everybody. Alright then, I'm off.'

Tatyana eventually managed to wash in the evening, after the last soldier left the tent under Petrenko's command.

Before leaving, the first sergeant left a pair of clean underwear for the girl – along with a towel, foot cloth, and laundry soap.

'And you? Tanya asked Maltsev, not seeing any fresh underwear for him.

'Just go ahead and wash yourselves. I'll do it later. Time is short: I have to get the typhoid case and poor Skvortsov to the battalion hospital. He's not out of the woods yet; head wounds are unpredictable.'

'When you return, the water will be cold, and it will be dark,' Tanya

said and got surprised herself with her unexpected insistence.

'You might be right,' the doctor's assistant agreed, and took off his tunic. 'It'll take me five minutes: head, neck, hands and arms. I'll wash up to my waist on my own.'

Pouring water from the pail onto the sergeant's soapy back, Tanya remembered Kucherenko's suspicious and caustic gaze. What he said seemed to make sense, but she also objected. He had spoken about vigilance and enemies of the people. But that just didn't apply to Maltsev.

After washing up, the doctor's assistant began to dry himself with a long towel. Tanya was looking at his broad, strong chest, and well-defined biceps on his arms. She couldn't easily tear her gaze away: men like that were only in the movies, she had thought.

That image stayed in Tatyana's mind as she washed and dressed and made her way along the familiar path to battalion HQ in the twilight.

The tent smelled of spirits. A clean-shaven officer, whom Tatyana didn't know, was holding a tin mug in his left hand and was about to drink the contents.

'A guest, a little pixie guest!' the officer put the mug aside. 'Who are you?'

'First Company Medical Instructor Rusakova,' Tatyana responded smartly.

The officer glanced questioningly at the battalion commander.

'She arrived yesterday and ran to the wounded right away. She helped Sedoy and had her baptism of fire,' Miroshnikov nodded approvingly at Tanya. 'And today she and the doctor's assistant were part of the sanitary treatment of the company. Where is Maltsev, by the way?'

Listening to the medical instructor's report, the battalion commander slowly rotated the mug on the lid of the barrel.

'Maltsev, you say, has headed off for the medical battalion, with two casualties. So, you can answer for him in his absence. What do you recommend against typhus, Comrade Medical Instructor?' Miroshnikov stared at Tanya and waited for an answer.

'Quarantine in the company, Comrade Major,' Tatyana began with confidence. 'Every day we'll perform preventive examinations, enforce the rules of hygiene, disinfect clothes, footwear, and—'

'My dear!' the battalion commander interrupted Tatyana with annoyance. 'Can you do all this in the trenches under fire? We cannot send the whole company to the rear! The only possible solution is quarantine.'

The battalion commander turned to Pichkhadze, who was sitting on a barrel, and said, 'Write up an order for quarantining the first company. No one visits them without my permission.'

The unknown officer glanced at Tanya and raised his tin mug. Then he said in rather a muffled voice, 'To you, to the battalion!'

Three mugs clashed loudly. The men drank a "front shot": a triple Only then did Tanya see that the unknown officer was missing his right hand. Noticing the girl's stare, he explained with a frown, 'A shell fragment carried it off along with my revolver.'

After a moment of silence, he added bitterly, 'I can shoot with my left hand – thank God! The hospital authorities forbade me from serving in combat and transferred me to the reserve. Over my dead body!'

'The battalion commissar killed four fascists in that battle. The Germans fled and began to mortar us,'

Miroshnikov recalled as he uncorked the flask and poured vodka into the mugs.

Just then, Petrenko ran into the dugout with a joyfully shouting, 'They have delivered!' He quickly saluted, grinning widely as he placed a package on the box, and reported, 'A truck with rations has arrived from the division. Bread, grain, sugar, stewed meat — twelve different items from the stores.'

Miroshnikov's face brightened up, 'How many portions per day?'

'I can't say, Comrade Major. The truck has just arrived and is being unloaded.'

'Give me the list!' the battalion commander smoothed the sheet of paper with a big red seal. 'Eight hundred kilogrammes of bread. That'll do for two days. As soon as you unload the truck, distribute half the bread to the men in the trenches, they're famished.'

The first sergeant saluted and left. Miroshnikov took a loaf of rye bread out of the package, turned it around and looked it over. Then he all but purred,

'It's not stale. Now we have got something to eat. We've been drinking on an empty stomach until now, like common drunks.'

The battalion commander cut off a big slice and held it out to Tatyana. Inhaling the smell of the fresh bread, Tanya felt delighted. While swallowing piece after piece, she felt as though she had never eaten anything more delicious.

Maltsev appeared in the dugout. His haggard look betrayed his exhaustion; he could barely stand.

'Sit down,' Miroshnikov said, moving aside and making room. 'Have a drink and a bite to eat. You can report later.'

'Good show, Sedoy!' the battalion commissar held a mug out to Maltsev. 'Cheers!'

'Congratulations on your return, Comrade Commissar!' the doctor's assistant said, and slowly drank the acrid spirit.

The officer drew a deep breath. 'My return!' he repeated ruefully. 'Tomorrow I'll be discharged. Commissar Vasilets' fighting days are over!'

They were silent for some time.

'Well, Sedoy,' the battalion commander interrupted the silence and moved aside the mugs brusquely. 'Go to the first company with the medical instructor. See if they are strictly observing the quarantine. In the morning you'll have a lot of trouble. The Germans are likely not to forgive yesterday's drubbing we gave them. Get ready for further attacks.'

Some unpleasant news was in store for Tanya and Maltsev.

'It looks like we've got another typhus case,' the company commander, a broad-chinned senior lieutenant, said with anxiety. Pavliuchenko, a gunner from the second platoon. 'He says he has a splitting headache and a fever.'

'Where is he now?' the doctor's assistant asked curtly.

Maltsev and Tanya found the gunner in the second platoon's trenches. He was sitting in the bottom of the ditch. He leaned against the earthen wall, his hands deep in the pockets of his greatcoat. The doctor's assistant put his hand on the man's forehead and noticed he was struggling to catch his breath.

'Your temperature, my friend, is high. Why didn't you tell us anything about it when you were examined in the tent?'

'I didn't have such a severe headache then.'

'Show me your tongue! Are you itchy anywhere?'

The gunner shook his head. Maltsev took a stethoscope out of his bag and began to sound the soldier's lungs.

'What's the matter with him?' the company commander asked as he jumped into the trench.

'Pneumonia, inflammation of the lungs. In the morning he'll be sent to the medical battalion. For now, he mustn't lie on the ground.'

'Ah, he's the best gunner we've got left!' the company commander waved his hand with annoyance. 'Where can we put him?'

The senior lieutenant looked at Tatyana, 'My soldiers have built a mud hut. It's better than any dugout. So maybe tonight...'

'Sure!' Tanya nodded. 'I'll go to battalion headquarters and spend the night in the storage room.'

'In a quarter of an hour it'll be pitch dark. I see no sense walking in darkness. You could easily lose your way,' the company commander objected. 'And it's going to rain soon.'

As if to confirm his words, raindrops began to patter on the leaves.

The patient was carried to the mud structure originally intended for the medical instructor. In the hut, the soldiers made a small table and a bench beside the bed, thickly covered with branches.

'It looks like a sanatorium, doesn't it?' the company commander joked, when the soldier, covered with two greatcoats and treated to sweet tea, closed his eyes in blissfully. 'Get well soon, gunner, and quickly, so the Germans won't miss you too much.'

Meanwhile, the rain intensified and soon covered the ground with quick-flowing rivulets.

'Please, come to my dugout,' invited the company commander, and led the doctor's assistant and Tanya after him towards two fallen pines.

The fir and pine branches covering the earthen floor filled the dugout with a distinct aroma. The little night light pushed the darkness into the corners of the dugout, lit the two bunks, and the small table between them.

'The more, the merrier,' the company commander pronounced in a pleased voice and shook the raindrops off his greatcoat. Seeing some confusion on Tanya's face, the officer waved his hand reassuringly, 'First we'll make you a private room. Help me please, Sedoy!'

Soon, two ground sheets were hung to the wire and fixed to the wooden ceiling. The plain construction divided the space in two.

'Doesn't it look like the Moscow-Sochi train?' the commander joked. 'Make yourselves at home, and I'll bring the mattresses.' It turned out that mattresses were four overcoats.

'After yesterday's scrap we got twenty spare ones. We didn't manage to carry them to the battalion storage,' the senior lieutenant's voice sounded gloomy this time.

'We should pray for the fallen, eh?'

The company commander looked at Maltsev and Tatyana questioningly. Without waiting for a response, he took a flask out of the kit, shook it and listened.

'It'll be enough for three drams,' he concluded, and broke the piece bread in three.

He rose from the bunk and stated, 'May our brave comrades rest in peace.' He took a sip and passed the flask to the doctor's assistant,

'I know you rarely drink. But on this occasion...'

Maltsev took a quick sip from the bottle and gave it to Tanya,

'Have a drink. There are only a few drops.'

'I know your name is Tanya,' the company commander said, screwing the flask cap back into place.

'I am Anatoly Zhelnov. Lay down and get yourself some sleep. The sergeant and I will sleep in the other bed. It won't bother us, we are used to anything.'

'And where do the men spend the night when it rains?' Tanya asked quickly and bit her lip, realizing that a question like that was out of place. The senior lieutenant stared at the girl, searched his pockets and took out a cigarette case. He lit one using the lamp and left the dugout.

The sleep claimed Tanya as soon as she lay on the bed, covered with a greatcoat and using her medical kit as a pillow. She didn't hear the company commander return, or how he lay down on the narrow bunk near the wall and answered her naive question in a quiet voice,

'It is a normal way to sleep in war. As for infantry

privates, bed is almost always a foxhole and a roll as a pillow, maybe a cloak too when it rains.'

Though Tanya's sleep was sound, she woke suddenly. She was having trouble breathing. There was a man's hand on her throat. Her heart began beating rapidly. The hand didn't move. Holding her breath, the girl carefully moved the hand to her shoulder.

'Tatyana Ivanovna, you are shameless girl!' her inner voice scolded. But to part with Sergey's hand! Tanya didn't doubt that the hand belonged to him. After a while, she dared to run her hand along his, thinking how kind and skillful he was. Sergey, who was lying on the opposite bunk, suddenly turned over, and the hand disappeared.

Tanya couldn't fall asleep. She heard Zhelnov and Maltsev coming and going, soldiers coming back with reports, and the senior lieutenant listening to them outside so as not to wake her.

When a sliver of morning sky penetrated into the dugout beneath the canvas flap spread across the entrance, Tatyana threw a greatcoat over her shoulders and went out. Not far away, Private Mishin was feeding Alma. Seeing Tanya, he waved hello. 'At last the division authorities have sent a team of dogs, but all four are females. Alma can't stand females. That's why I have to feed them separately,' the guide said with regret.

'What kind of females?' Tanya asked without thinking.

'The team of dogs was sent from the division to evacuate and transport the wounded. And all of them are females. Alma would get on with male dogs easily.'

'Do dogs really take wounded men to the medical battalion and…'

'Not to the medical battalion. They drag the wounded off the battlefield on a little drag sledge.'

'How does that work?' Tanya asked with doubt in her voice.

'Like this: the dogs run up to the wounded soldier and stop. The soldier does his best to turn over onto the sledge, and the dogs drag him to our trenches. When it's dark there's no alternative to them. They can smell where the wounded are.'

Looking at Alma as she licked her breakfast, the guide hurried on, 'Well, I'm going to the forest. I tied four dogs to a tree and now I have to feed them.'

Zhelnov came up to the dugout with quick steps and greeted Tanya warmly,

'How did you sleep?' Without waiting for an answer, he informed her, 'Maltsev left for the medical platoon. We need more medication. Regimental reconnaissance has shown that there is movement along the German front. You may walk to the bog, and to the tent. There is some water in the barrels, but it got cold overnight. You can wash yourself there. Once you're back we can have breakfast.'

'I'd like to visit the patient with pneumonia.'

'Rogov took him to the medical battalion in a cart.' Zhelnov furrowed his brows and said anxiously, 'We have got a lot to do today. By the way, can you shoot?' Tatyana shook her head.

'We'll teach you. A medical instructor near the front has to be armed.'

Porridge with a whiff of meat was served for breakfast

again. After the meal, the company commander led Tanya along the trenches of the platoon strong points.

'Keep low here, two snipers are working on the other side,' warned Zhelnov, moving along the narrow trench.

Many soldiers welcomed the familiar girl with a nod or a wave of a hand. Some winked good-naturedly and joked harmlessly.

'The company sector is about one kilometre long,' Zhelnov announced to Tatyana, when they reached the edge of the last trench, that of the third platoon.

'We gather the wounded in the ravine near the bog and the tent, where you and Maltsev examined and disinfected the men. When the enemy attacks we'll suffer casualties of course. You'll give first aid here in the trenches. After the attack has been beaten off you and the medical orderlies drag the wounded to the ravine and the tent. Then you provide further transportation to get them to the medical battalion.'

'And if we attack?'

'An excellent question,' Zhelnov looked at Tatyana with approval. 'We won't attack. We have nobody and nothing to attack with. There are only a hundred soldiers left in the company, and three light machine guns. We've got almost no grenades. The day before yesterday we had twelve machine guns, but in the past two days the Germans killed nine gun teams with mortar fire.'

After a pause, he said decisively, 'But we will counter-attack, if the fascists reach our lines. The Germans are weak in bayonet fighting. When they retreat, you and the medical orderlies move forward behind our men.

Watch where the wounded soldiers fall and treat them. Is everything clear?'

'Yes, it is, Comrade Senior Lieutenant!' Tanya answered according to regulations. 'Permission to carry out orders?'

'What exactly are you going to do?' the company commander asked.

'I'll ask the soldiers if they have complaints. If necessary, I'll examine them. And we must prepare a spot for the wounded in the ravine.'

'You understand our situation well, Rusakova. I'll send two orderlies to set up the casualty area. They'll bring greatcoats. The wounded shouldn't lie on the bare ground.'

Tatyana didn't manage to ask the soldiers anything. Just then a fearsome howl split the air.

'Get down!' the senior lieutenant thundered, and threw the medical instructor on the grass, wet after the night rain.

The German shells burst near and far, sometimes throwing dirt on Zhelnov and Tanya as they lay side-by-side.

'Short dashes to the hut!' the company commander shouted into Tanya's ear. 'As soon as the fire stops, run back to the men's position!'

In the hut, Tanya shook the dirt from her hair as the bursts continued.

'What if some of our men are wounded?' she thought, forgetting her fear.

Once the firing stopped, Tanya sprinted the hundred

metres to the first platoon's position. She jumped in, medical kit in hand.

'God has shown mercy for the moment, we all seem to be alive,' a tall soldier told her, looking with delight at the fair-haired beauty who seemed to have descended from the heavens. 'The second platoon has gotten the short end of the stick. The Germans are pounding their position. You'd better wait here for a while...'

Tatyana stopped listening and rushed along the trench to the second platoon. In the first traverse a frightful scene met her eyes: a soldier lay on his back, his face covered in blood. His ear was quivering, nearby lay a part of his leg. The soldier was convulsing: he groaned and clawed at the earth with his hands. Tatyana hesitated for a second or two: help this one in his agony or to go on and save those who could be saved. She took a tourniquet from the bag and tightened it around the bleeding limb. 'Time," she thought. She wrote "7:00" in pencil on a bit of paper and pushed it under the tourniquet.

Someone jumped into the trench. Tatyana turned around. Mishin, covered with dirt, saluted, 'Don't you need a dog's help?'

'I'll take any help I can get. Hold his hands!'

Tanya began to wipe the blood off the soldier's face.

'I saw you in Lomakin's foxhole and slithered over to you. Wow! He wasn't lucky! The shell seems to burst nearby. Might have been the last one. The Germans look to have stopped firing.'

Having cleaned the face of the wounded soldier, Tatyana sighed with relief.

'The shell fragments are small. He may survive.'

Bandaging the soldier, she said sternly to Mishin, 'He must be sent to the medical battalion immediately. They can save him there.'

'I understand, Comrade Tatyana! I've got a four dog-power vehicle just for that.'

Cupping his hands, the guide made a loud sound like the hoot of an owl. Soon, near the foxhole, the team of dogs appeared. Mishin and Tanya put the wounded soldier onto a sledge.

Tatyana nodded and hurried along the narrow, zig-zagging trench. Suddenly she remembered that she hadn't injected the soldier with antitetanic serum. She jumped out of the trench and rushed after the team of dogs that had disappeared into the shrubs.

When she came back, she saw a familiar broad-shouldered figure in the trench. She felt glad Sergey had returned.

Without realizing what she was doing, Tanya jumped into the ditch and wrapped her arms around him. Maltsev gently smoothed the girl's tousled hair, straightened her field cap, which had been knocked askew, and said with barely restrained emotion, 'We must go, Tanya, there are many wounded men.'

There were also many dead. The Germans had plastered the 300-metre section of the second platoon with shells. Mishin and his dogs dragged two badly-wounded soldiers to the ravine and laid them on greatcoats. Soon the medicine the doctor's assistant had brought from the battalion medical station ran out. Tanya's medical kit was also empty.

'I took the last bandage!' Tanya shouted to Maltsev in despair, while she was bandaging a soldier with a chest wound.

'Can your dogs get to battalion headquarters?' the sergeant asked Mishin, who had stopped the team of dogs at the edge of the trench.

'These ones don't know the way yet. Alma will surely get there, we've been at the headquarters more than once.'

Having wiped the blood off his hands, the doctor's assistant tied the empty medical kits together with straps. He took a pen out of his pocket and wrote on one of them: "We need medicine. Maltsev." Then he gave the kit to the guide.

Mishin tied the team of dogs to a tree in the ravine. Then he took twenty steps and shouted: 'Alma! To me!'

He fastened the medical kits to the dog's back and took Alma to the path which led to battalion HQ. Then he clearly repeated the following words three times: 'Run to the post!'

Wagging her tail, the dog ran off into the sparse growth of trees. Alma stuck doggedly to the path in the high grass that had begun to grow yellow at the end of summer. Maltsev gathered field dressings from the bodies of the dead and gave some to Tanya.

'How many lightly wounded are there?' Zhelnov asked as he jumped into the trench.

'I'm bandaging the ninth,' the doctor's assistant answered.

'All of them remain in the line!' the company commander decided.

'We can't hold out otherwise: of thirty-four soldiers only five were not hit.'

'You are also wounded!' Tanya exclaimed, seeing blood on the senior lieutenant's face.

'It's nothing Just a scratch, not a wound!'

'It's not a trifle,' Maltsev said after he'd cleaned the commander's bloody temple. 'Shell fragments often infect wounds. Let's wipe the wound with vodka,' he added, looking at a flask on the senior lieutenant's belt.

While Tanya was bandaging the company commander's head, the doctor's assistant walked along the positions of the platoon and ordered the lightly wounded soldiers to stay at their posts.

The distant noise of engines filled the air with anxious expectation of the coming danger.

'Two tanks are approaching,' Zhelnov said angrily as he looked through his binoculars. 'Looks like Panzer I's – the machine-gun infantry support tank. But we have nothing to counter them with.'

The company commander opened his eyes wide and yelled at the soldier sitting in the nearest him, 'Simagin! Run to battalion HQ and don't come back without an antitank rifle.'

Simagin shot up and out of the trench like a bolt, one hand holding down his field cap.

Zhelnov glanced at Tanya and rubbed his chin. Then he said, 'Your place now is with the wounded, in the ravine. They must be taken to the regimental medical station as soon as possible by any means.'

'Can I stay with you?' Tanya looked at the company commander pleadingly.

'No, you can't! There are only fifteen of us here. Maltsev can cope alone.'

Leaving the trench, Tanya looked back and gasped with surprise: in the distance little figures, which looked like living toys, were following the German tanks. There were many of them, and they were running across the same field where Tatyana had seen her first action.

Mishin was sitting near the tent and doing something with the sledge. Seeing the medical instructor, the soldier smiled, 'At last! Two soldiers are getting worse, they are groaning all the time.'

Tanya examined the wounded in the ravine and understood that those two needed help urgently. She quickly asked Mishin, 'Is it far from here to the regiment aid station?'

'Three kilometres.'

'These two soldiers must be evacuated without delay.'

'It'll be hard for the dogs, they probably won't manage to drag two men,' Mishin said doubtfully.

Knitting his brows, he thought a minute and then waved his hand,

'Well, I'll join them, we'll deliver them together.'

The German tanks were clearly headed towards the second platoon's position. The noise of their engines grew more and more distinct. The wounded soldiers began fidgeting anxiously.

'The company commander said that the tanks just had machine guns,' Tanya said to calm their nerves.

'Makes no difference,' a soldier with a bandaged head said gloomily. 'They will crush us here like bugs.'

The rattling of the machine guns now mingled with the noise of the engines, followed by sharp report of rifle fire. Then several loud explosions followed one upon the other.

'The fascists are throwing grenades,' a soldier, wounded in both legs, observed gloomily. 'And our boys haven't got any, we used them all yesterday.'

Alma slipped into the ravine like a shadow. Two bulging medical kits and another sack were tied to her back and the sides. She ran up to Tatyana.

'A clever dog you are!' Tanya exclaimed happily. 'Let's get to the trenches!'

Tanya ran the three hundred metres to the lines as bullets whistled past, clipping the pine branches around her. Seeing the company commander in a foxhole, she rolled head over heels to the trench. Spreading her paws wide, Alma landed near her.

'What have you got in the sack?' the senior lieutenant asked briefly.

Shrugging her shoulders, Tanya began to free the dog from the load. The sack turned out to be so heavy that she could hardly lift it.

'Hand grenades! Antitank shells! Six of them! Machine gun ammo!'

Zhelnov cried out joyfully.

'Good, Alma! Now hold on, bastards!'

Patting the dog's head, he ordered Tatyana, 'Find Maltsev, he is somewhere over on the right side in one of the foxholes. Give him a medical kit and two grenades.'

Tanya found Sergey quickly. Kneeling in the foxhole, he was winding a bandage around a branch. Next to him stood a tin with some liquid.

'Grenades!' the doctor's assistant shouted. 'And I was just preparing a Molotov cocktail. Now we'll fight them off.'

Looking into Tanya's eyes, he said urgently, 'Crawl back to the ravine, and be quick!'

Tanya shook her head. Danger was approaching the defenders of the platoon strong point, and she couldn't leave Sergey.

'Go! Now!' the doctor's assistant shouted, but just at the same moment he grabbed the belt of her tunic and dragged her roughly to the bottom of the trench.

The guns of the approaching tanks began to throw lead against the parapet of the trench. In response, Zhelnov's gun began firing in short bursts, and the rifle fire of the men started to crackle. As if meeting an unexpected obstacle, the lines of attackers lay down, but the armoured vehicles kept on moving towards the trenches.

'The bastard's coming right at us!' Maltsev shouted, raising his head over the edge of the trench for a second.

'Lie down on the bottom!' he cried to Tatyana. 'And don't get up!'

Grabbing a grenade, the doctor's assistant hurled it towards the approaching German tank with all his might.

The explosion of the hand grenade, which fell short the target, raised a cloud of dirt and debris into the air, briefly obscuring the view of the crew.

The second grenade damaged a track, and the tank slowly began to whirl around. The company commander's machine fell silent. The German infantry resumed the attack, gathering behind the second tank, which was crawling towards the parapet of the front trench. Two antitank grenades boomed nearby. They forced the German infantry to go to ground again, but the tank kept on moving. Rolling awkwardly over the parapet, it crawled alongside the trench and started to run fire on the foxholes.

Leaning into the wall of the trench, Tanya bit her lips in helpless fury. She thought bitterly, 'I'm sitting here like a fool! Sergey is fighting the Germans, and I can't even shoot.'

The clatter of tracks and the roar of an engine made her look up. Tanya saw a black and white cross on the side of the tank and a big number "13" on the turret. Acrid exhaust fumes surrounded her.

Just then the whitish cloud of the tank's exhaust was disturbed by the figure of the doctor's assistant. He jumped up from the foxhole in a flash and rushed after the tank as it moved on. Tanya saw him holding a tin to his chest as he ran. In his other hand, a burning torch cut the air in rhythm with his leaping bounds. She saw Sergey catch up with the tank, break the petrol-filled bottle against its armour, and fall suddenly, hitting the ground still holding the burning torch.

Obeying an unknown force, Tanya jumped out of the trench and rushed towards the spot where he had fallen. Bullets were whistling past her, but none found its mark. She managed to grab the torch and throw it at the tank as it began to turn around. The last thing Tanya saw was a column of fire burst upwards from the machine.

The bullet entered her back beneath the shoulder blade and felt like a sharp needle-prick. She lost consciousness, fell to the ground, and did not see how the reinforcements that arrived used an anti-tank gun to silence the German tank's guns, or how with a short and furious bayonet attack into the enemy flank the first platoon forced the Germans to retreat whence they'd come.

She neither saw nor felt how Mishin and Rogov carefully put her on a cart, along with Sergey and four other wounded soldiers, and how diligently Mashka quickly took them to the divisional medical battalion.

Somewhere nearby, drops of water were periodically hitting the bottom of a tin. The sound echoed painfully in Tatyana's consciousness. She tried to focus and see clearly, but couldn't. She tried to turn her head towards the sound but couldn't: a sharp pain cut through her back.

'Don't you turn over, the drain will fall out,' a woman's confident and quiet voice sounded nearby. 'You need a bedpan, don't you?'

Tatyana's thighs felt the chill of the metal.

'Do go ahead,' the same voice continued. 'It's time to come to. It's the fifth day, isn't it?'

Before Tatyana's eyes there appeared a fuzzy figure in

white. 'Where am I?' she asked.

'In the field hospital.'

The figure tucked in the blanket and carefully took out the bedpan. Then Tanya was warned by a strict voice.

'Lie quietly, you mustn't move now. I'll soon come back and give you something to eat.'

The drops kept on pinging against the tin at even intervals. It seemed to Tanya that someone had put a chisel to her head and was hammering on it. Little by little, the sounds began to lose their intensity. The drops fell less and less frequently.

Sergey's image appeared suddenly with a grenade in his hand. Then the German tank appeared, wreathed in flames, but the vision only lasted a second before Tatyana was claimed by sleep's silent embrace.

She didn't hear the telephone ringing, people walking nearby, men's voices arguing. She only woke up when someone wiped her face with a wet towel.

'You are awake. Good.'

The deep voice belonged to a stout woman in a white smock with bulging pockets. She raised Tanya's head with her plump palm and took an egg from her pocket. She cracked it against something hard and pronounced sympathetically, 'Drink a bit, my dear. We have no salt, so you'll have to swallow it as it is.'

Another egg appeared from the same pocket. But Tanya was tired, and with a weak move of her hand she tried to refuse it.

'Alright, rest a little,' the woman said and began to tell Tanya the following.

'In our village, Khmeleuka, there is a hospital now. Some of the houses had boarded up windows, because so many people had been evacuated east. All the men had been mobilized. Why should the houses stand empty? The wounded soldiers need treatment. So, our village women joined the hospital crew and work as caretakers, nurses, we wash linen and underwear, and mend uniforms as well. There are nearly two hundred wounded soldiers and officers at the hospital now. Each house is packed with them, and they need nursing. The hospital doctors cannot manage without us.'

Feeding Tanya the second egg, the woman took a clay pot and an aluminum spoon.

'Eat some sour cream. The head doctor, Sokolov, ordered me to feed you well.'

Swallowing some spoonfuls of home-made sour cream, Tanya leaned back on the pillow in exhaustion.

'Well, I am leaving now,' the nurse said, becoming serious. 'In the next house there are wounded soldiers, I'm off to take care of them. And you: sleep and recover.' Then she smiled and added, 'My name is Katerina.'

Quite nearby someone began to turn the handle of a telephone. Tanya opened her eyes and carefully turned her head towards the sounds. Her gaze got no further than a curtain made of sheets. Suddenly a hand pulled the curtain aside.

'How are you feeling, Comrade Medical Instructor?' the sympathetic voice of the tall man in a white overall asked. 'Do you know where you are?'

'In hospital' Tanya whispered with difficulty.

'Don't talk. Answer with your eyes. Right, you are now in an army field hospital, and I am Doctor Boris Aleksandrovich Sokolov. I'm in charge around here. Just now the senior surgeon is on the telephone. He'll examine you as soon as he is free. Our hospital is located in a village, spread amongst thirty houses. This one is the headquarters. You are the only female patient we have and we can't treat you in the same room as the men, so we decided to put you here. You have one job: to recover as soon as possible. Medical personnel are like gold to us. There should be eight doctors on the hospital staff, but in fact there are only two of us. We badly need medical personnel. Do you understand?'

Tanya dropped her eyes.

'There is one more thing. Everything that happens behind this curtain doesn't concern you. No rumours or gossip. in a word, keep quiet.'

Suddenly, the telephone receiver slammed loudly. Drawing the curtain, the boss stepped back into the room. There he asked the telephone operator, 'And, will they allot us anything? What did the brass promise?'

'The army stores are empty. The frontline stores are empty as well. He said that everything had been sent to the south. But yesterday Moscow received a shipment of medical supplies via lend-lease. So they can give us something. The boss phoned the highest authorities and they've approved. But we've got to get it soon. If we are late, it will be transported to the centre. In that case we'll get it in two – or three-weeks' time and it won't be much then.'

'There have been four fatal cases in the last day and night alone. Gangrene, sepsis, suppurative infections.'

'We have another thirty just like them,' said the head physician, his voice trembling in despair. 'There are no sulfa drugs, not a single pill. How can we treat anything? How?'

Struck by what she had heard, Tanya thought of the wounded soldiers lying in the village houses, whose lives hung in the balance due to the lack of medical supplies. Trying to over, she groaned in pain. Almost at the same time a man in a white coat appeared. Removing his glasses, the man turned to Tanya, examined the wound on her back and nodded his head with satisfaction, 'It's coming along well. Tomorrow we'll remove the drain, and in a week you'll be dancing the polka and the fox trot.'

'Back in the field with wounded, syringe in hand,' the hospital boss commented gloomily.

'By the way, the situation with syringes is also catastrophic, we only have four left,' the head physician said quietly.

'How can that be? Who broke them?'

'Simagina couldn't handle a wounded soldier. The patient lashed out and broke the syringe while unconscious.'

'We'll soon be in such a state ourselves, Gennady Matveevich. Inform all the nurses again that they will answer for such cases with their lives,' the head of the hospital said with a note of irritation.

The door flew open. A military man with three cubes on red collar tabs appeared. The doctors left Tanya and went to meet him.

'What's the situation, Donchenko? Report.' The hospital boss sat down heavily on the wide bench that stood near the window.

The red-haired officer with prominent cheekbones spoke rapidly, furrowing his white eyebrows, 'There will be no hot food for dinner today, Comrade Doctor. We just can't manage it. You didn't allow us to kill Zuyeva's cow. There are eight hens in the village, but we need them...'

'What about Zinaida Polyakova's goat?' the head of the hospital interrupted. 'You wanted to talk to her this morning and try to convince her.'

'Yes, I tried everything. I reminded her that she had a son at the front. But she refused! She's already given the wounded all the potatoes and beetroots she had stored for winter. She says without the goat she will die of starvation.'

'Where is her son serving? What front?'

'In the air force. He is a navigator, according to the villagers.'

'According to the villagers...you're not only my logistics assistant, but the area commandant as well. You must know everything.'

The hospital chief rose from the bench and walked slowly alongside the table which stood near the wall. The table was covered with embroidered ruchniks.8 He turned to the logistics assistant and sighed, 'So, the wounded men will have clear soup again.'

'And two hundred grams of bread for dinner,' the red-haired officer hurriedly added, and would have continued

---

8   Traditional East Slavic towel or cloth.

but for the angry stare of his superior.

'I hope you understand that we are in grave danger. In two weeks, the wounded will begin to suffer from dystrophy and scurvy with this food. Without proper meals the body's resistance against infections is precisely none. It means that soldiers can't even think about returning to the front. Mortality will no doubt increase significantly,' the doctor reminded him.

'I'm doing my best, Comrade Doctor, but our requests are not being fulfilled,' the captain said gloomily. 'A soldier needs nine hundred grams of bread a day, but we only get four hundred. We don't receive grain regularly and when they do send some it's half of what we need.'

'You are not doing everything that can be done, Comrade Donchenko! Yes, the fascists occupied Kuban, the granary of our country, and they've reached the Volga. It's clear that those fighting on that front get priority. But even if that's the case, you must find other solutions. Sit down and write down my orders.'

The hospital chief paused, and began to dictate while pacing restlessly, 'From now on, all lightly wounded soldiers will be sent to the nearest forest to gather mushrooms, berries and medicinal herbs every day. All personnel who are not busy taking care of the wounded are to join the forest team. All wounded and hospital staff are to receive a daily ration of pine decoction, three hundred grams per person.'

There came a loud and insistent knocking at the door of the house. The hospital chief stopped speaking and faced the door. Then he said in a cold biting voice, 'Come in!'

An elderly woman wrapped in a home-made woolen kerchief, stepped across the threshold, heavily leaning heavily on a knotted stick. The red-haired logistics assistant left a fat inkblot on the sheet of paper. He jumped up and stared at the woman with wide-open eyes.

'I am Zinaida Polyakova. I've brought a goat, Sonka is her name. It's for the wounded men.'

The old woman's voice trembled. The hospital head stood stock still in surprise. The senior surgeon turned to the window, took out a kerchief from his pocket and pressed it to his eyes. Behind the curtain, Tanya cried silently and buried her head in the pillow.

'The goat is here, it's tied near the entrance.'

The woman bowed purposefully, opened the door and descended the creaking steps of the porch. Donchenko made to rush after her, but the hospital head stopped him, saying, 'Let her be. Let her say her farewells to the goat. And one more thing. Take her on as a nurse.'

'She has an injured leg, Comrade Doctor, she won't be able...'

'She is the mother of a pilot. She'll do what she can. Put the order through and put her on the payroll.'

The hospital chief smashed his fist on the table, 'And I order you to feed the wounded men of this hospital at any cost!'

Then he addressed Donchenko, 'Prepare orders for both ambulances. One of them we'll send to Moscow for medical supplies. The other will have to bring back some food. Think where we might be able to find some. Send it eastwards, to the rear. I don't care if it has to go 500 kilometres from here. The collective farms there surely have something. Meet with the authorities, ask and demand. God damn it! Don't come back without food.'

'Yes, Sir!'

The logistics assistant wiped his sweaty forehead with his sleeve and made to leave.

'Wait! Take this message to the senior nurse in the Tent Four.'

The head doctor wrote some words on a piece of paper, folded it over and handed it to the captain. 'Dismissed. Do your best!'

The red-haired officer left in a rush, the door banging shut behind him.

'Take a seat and come closer, Gennady Matveevich,' the head doctor said to the senior surgeon, 'We have to compose a request for medical supplies. We should ask for a minimum. The chap in charge of the medical services for our front area warned me that if we ask for too much, we won't get anything at all.'

'But we need practically everything! Surgical instruments like scissors, forceps, syringes, needles, and medical gloves. The ether ran out last week. Novocaine, rivanol, streptocide, sulfidine, and codeine. We have no iodine either. I could list the things we need all day.'

'A day, you say?' the head doctor scoffed and looked sternly at his counterpart. 'In two hours, our ambulance leaves for Moscow, and must arrive at the central warehouse there before the end of the day.'

There was confusion in the round eyes of the head surgeon.

'Boris Aleksandrovich, we can't get there before nightfall! It's nearly four hundred kilometres. And half of that is on a dirt road.'

'It's won't be easy, of course. But our wounded men are dying, that's why I consider getting these supplies our utmost priority. I hope you share my plan to solve this problem. By the way, Captain Donchenko will be sent to Moscow, not you.'

The senior surgeon started in surprise and glanced at his superior, not understanding what he meant.

'Precisely. Not you, Gennady Matveevich. Anything can happen on the road, and if I stay here alone, you see, I can't do much for two hundred patients. A single soldier can't win a battle.'

'But Donchenko…' the doctor started, and shrugged his shoulders.

'Make up a list of the required medication, Gennady Matveevich. Captain Donchenko will be accompanied by a medical man as a consultant.'

'Who is that man?' the physician asked as he fastened his eyes upon the calm face of his superior.

'You'll see, he'll soon be here.'

Shaking his head doubtfully, the physician began to write up the request. The house was filled with silence. Against the background of a scratching pen, Tatyana's blurry thoughts ranged far and wide. The last of these haunted her as she fell asleep: 'What's become of Sergey?'

The door of the house swung open with a knock.

'Oh, here is our doctor now, he's easy to find,' the head of the hospital announced with a pleased smile. 'Sit down, Comrade Doctor's Assistant.'

On glancing at the person who had just entered the room, the head surgeon tousled his grey hair, and said 'Boris Aleksandrovich, Maltsev has a cracked rib. He will have to stay here at least a week…how can we send him? He won't stand ten hours shaking in a truck!'

'Desperate times call for desperate measures, Gennady Matveevich. Maltsev is an experienced doctor. I convinced the army medical command to include him on their staff, and they'll make it official soon. So, we're all colleagues here.'

The hospital chief briefly explained the situation and held out a sheet of paper, folded in four: 'If there's a problem, call this number. They'll help you.'

After a pause, he put his hand on Sergey's shoulder and said, 'I'm sending you, even though you're not fully healed. I take the blame for that, but there's no other way. Delivering our papers to Moscow is an important task, but to get the medicine we need so badly is much more difficult. You'll see that once you reach your destination. The names of the medication are in Latin, the instructions and the technical descriptions of the equipment are in English, which you can speak. Who else can read them but you? By the way, how do you know English?'

'My father taught me. He was a philologist, a professor.'

The head of the hospital looked aside. Frowning, he pronounced quietly,

'I understand your problem. As soon as you get back, we'll have a talk. Is the mission clear?'

'Yes, it is, Comrade Doctor!' Sergey saluted. 'Permission to leave?'

'Donchenko will receive our application for the medical supplies. A straw mattress must be put in the back of the truck for you to lie on. Don't forget to take a flask with tea, and some bread. Get going!'

The cool September sun reached its zenith as the truck, covered with a tent, left the field hospital the small Valdai village Khmelevka. Dirty water splashed up from the ruts in the track as the truck rolled slowly to the east.

The mattress, packed with straw, dulled the effects of the shaking somewhat, but the wound in Maltsev's side pained him with each pothole. Sergey had to lean on his arms to lessen the shock to his body as the truck swayed and lurched to and fro.

Suddenly the truck began to slow down, and then stopped. Danchenko's red-haired head looked into the back.

'Get out, Maltsev! Get into the cab, it's a little smoother. I'm afraid you won't make it.' Deftly jumping into the back, the captain joked, 'We don't need any fatalities on the way.'

Sergey gave him a thankful look and carefully got down from the truck. The driver, a big-boned middle-aged soldier, seemed to be glad of the change. He rolled a cigarette and began to tell Sergey about the virtues of the truck that was bravely overcoming the pitted road.

'This truck is a relentless worker. After Torzhok we'll go along the highway, so I'll get it up to a speed of seventy kilometres.'

Sergey looked at the speedometer. It showed about thirty kilometres per hour.

'I'll get it up!' the driver repeated with confidence, when he noticed the glance of the sergeant. 'I drove a truck like this for nine years before the war. This one came to the hospital in spring. It's a wartime model, because there are metal and parts shortages now.

Sergey noticed that the door of the cab was made of wood and canvas.

'The left headlight is being fixed now at the plant. And there only two wheels on the back axle, not four like before the war,' the driver told Sergey. 'So you can't load a tonne and a half on it...it would get stuck right away on a road like this.'

Once they'd reached the slope of a hill, the talkative driver stopped the truck. 'Time to feed the "horse."'

He pushed his cap back on his forehead, jumped out of the cab and swiftly opened the bonnet. Soon the truck "fed" from the jerry can and began moving again.

'The tank holds forty litres, enough for two hundred kilometres, not more,' the soldier explained. 'But kerosene can also be used once the engine is warm. In the hospital stores there is no petrol, but there are three full barrels of kerosene.'

A droning in the sky, sprinkled with cumulus clouds, did not perturb the driver.

When he saw Sergey's concerned look, he waved his hand nonchalantly,

'Friendly planes. Our aerodrome is only thirty kilometres away, just behind the wood, so they...'

The canvas cab began shaking, pummelled by fists from its passenger in the back.

'Maslovsky!' Donchenko shouted wildly from the back. 'Put the brakes on, you devil! Everyone run to the wood!'

'Brakes, brakes!' the driver grumbled.

Suddenly he rolled out of the cab in one motion, broke through the roadside hedge, and rushed into the thick spruce thicket. The logistics assistant followed right behind him. Sergey flung open the cabin door and looked up. About 500 metres up, two German "Stuka" aircraft flew westwards.

'They have finished their bombing run and are returning to base,' Sergey thought as he stepped on the footboard of the truck. An acute pain shot through his back. He only had enough strength to get out of the cab and sit on the ground near the front bumper. Both the planes descended and flew just over the earth road.

Their silhouettes approached faster and faster, with their distinct curved wings and fixed landing gear. Sergey closed his eyes and felt goosebumps rise all over his body. The captain shouted from the forest through the thick branches:

'Maltsev! Why on earth are you sitting there!? Get over here!'

Having filled the forest with a mighty roar, the planes began to disappear in the distance.

'It's over!' Sergey sighed with relief and put his hand to his forehead, covered with perspiration.

The angry barking of a machine gun made him

tremble. Then silence came. He knew it was silent because he could hear the subtle hum of the mosquitoes.

'What's the matter with you, Maltsev? Are you wounded?' asked Donchenko, who appeared nearby.

'It's alright,' Sergey leaned on the bumper and tried to rise. The captain's face reddened. He helped the doctor's assistant handstand up. Helping him to the cab, he let out a frustrated sigh and muttered with confusion, 'More trouble. You seemed to be walking. How did I...? Everything is turning out badly...'

'The back end of the truck is shot up, the left set of wheels have been shot through,' Maslovsky said gravely and rolled the spare wheel. 'Now if we hit some nail or something else...we'll have to stop.'

In a quarter of an hour the truck began to move again.

'The rear gunner got us as they pulled away,' the driver commented in an expert tone and exhaled his cigarette smoke towards Sergey. 'It looks like he had some cartridges left. When we took some wounded pilots to the hospital, I heard that the Germans use the airport in Demyansk to bomb Yaroslavl, Uglich, and Rybinsk. And they even bombed Gorky. They make me sick!'

'When will we get to Moscow?' Sergey asked, wanting to change the topic.

'It depends,' Maslovsky flicked his cigarette butt to the side of the road. 'We'll get there by evening, if the skies don't trouble us any more. You should have a rest, Comrade Doctor's Assistant.'

He put his hands on the steering wheel and began

to quietly whistle a familiar tune. Rocking slightly, engine droning resolutely, the truck overcame the next slope. The driver carefully charted course around the holes and slowed down to negotiate the numerous ruts and rough patches.

Sergey tried to forget what had happened half an hour earlier and to persuade himself that both of his companions had done the right thing.

'If they had carried me to the forest, all of us might have bought it, and then…' he thought. He didn't want to think of how it could have ended.

Sergey was tired from the driving. His eyelids got heavier and heavier, and eventually closed. He plunged into a deep slumber.

He woke up because the truck stopped, and Donchenko was standing on the running board pulling at the sleeve of his tunic.

'Let's change places. Soon we'll reach Kalinin, and our documents will be checked there.'

Sergey got into the back of the truck again and settled down on the soft mattress, which smelled of straw. On the road, covered with crushed stones, the truck shook much less, and it began to pick up the pace.

The team arrived in Moscow as the late summer setting sun painted the rooves of the houses crimson. The houses lined gloomy streets which bristled with antitank "hedgehog" obstacles.

At the warehouses of the General Military Medical Administration, work was in full swing. The lieutenant colonel of the quartermaster's service, a tall blond with a trimmed moustache and a soft round face, quickly looked through the application documents, shrugged his shoulders and pronounced in surprise,

'Who sent you here?'

'The head of the hospital telephoned General Shamov, who promised...'

'Shamov, you say?' the officer stared at Donchenko. 'Well, the Doctor Shamov is here. We'll ask him and clarify your problem.' Looking at Sergey, who was standing off to the side, he asked, 'Who is this?'

'Our doctor's assistant,' answered Donchenko, who had immediately included Maltsev in the hospital staff. 'He is our team medical consultant. He knows English well.'

Scrutinising Sergey, the lieutenant-colonel ordered, 'Both of you, follow me!'

In the large warehouse, shelves and stands were full of boxes, metal barrels, sacks, multicoloured bundles and packages of every description. Some of them lay in the passages, which were populated by people in blue overalls moving with surprising agility. Each pile of boxes was tipped deftly onto a two-wheeled cart and sped over to the large sliding doors at the loading dock.

In the centre of the building, near some unpacked boxes, a lean soldier in spectacles was attentively examining a bottle he had just taken out of a bag. A woman next to him was explaining something to him and gesticulating with her hands. People in uniforms were sitting at two big tables looking into some thick books from time to time. They wrote something in big note-books. Girls with military jackets on their shoulders were typing. Two soldiers were opening a large wooden box with hammers.

The lieutenant-colonel gestured to his guests to wait and went up to the military man in spectacles. He saluted and said something quietly.

Seeing three golden rhombi on his collar, Donchenko and Sergey stood at attention and, being given a sign to approach, did so with parade-ground steps.

'Your boss phoned me and reported on the situation,' the military doctor said. He furrowed his bushy brows and quickly looked through the hospital's application. Then he returned the papers to Donchenko and looked at Sergey,

'I've been told you know English. Excellent. Do you see how much medical equipment the US has sent? The first shipment from Arkhangelsk has reached us. We've been studying the manuals and instructions for a day and a half; our translators can hardly cope.'

The doctor turned his head towards the people who were sitting at the tables. 'And you are a medical man, you'll help them to manage more quickly. By the way, what high school did you graduate from?'

'The First Leningrad Institute, Therapeutic Faculty, Comrade Doctor.'

'How long have you been at the front?'

'Since July 1941.'

The doctor raised his thick eyebrows, which turned his forehead into a labyrinth of wrinkles.

'Why do you have the rank of assistant? Why not a doctor? Why aren't you an officer? Did you do something wrong? You got demoted?' the doctor sounded angry as he spat the questions.

Sergey was silent: he was looking at the lieutenant colonel, Donchenko, and the unfamiliar woman. He did not want to answer the questions in their presence.

The military doctor understood, and suggested unexpectedly in English, 'Say it in English, then'

'My father, Professor Maltsev, was found guilty of anti-Soviet activity and imprisoned in 1937. He was sentenced to a ten-year term, according to Article 58, Paragraph 2,' Sergey said in a muted voice.

The doctor rubbed his chin with his long, thin fingers. 'Where is your father now?'

'I don't know,' Sergey responded, his voice trembling. 'He was sentenced without the right to correspondence.'

The doctor took out a snow-white handkerchief from his pocket, took off his glasses and began to wipe them. 'I'll try to find out something about your father and then inform you. And now get to work. We'll give your hospital medication and first-aid materials, as much as we can,' the doctor announced and put on his glasses.

Looking at Sergey, he said, 'And your English is good. In 1913 I mastered it quite well, when I worked at William Mayo's clinic in Minnesota. But I've forgotten it since then. Many of my colleges can speak German, but there is no one to speak English with. But we have no time for that now. Alright then, time to get down to business.'

The doctor nodded to Sergey, then had a short conversation with the lieutenant colonel and made his way to the translators' tables.

'General Shamov has decided you are to be given 50 % of the requested materials,' the lieutenant-colonel announced to Donchenko. 'Take into account that we are trying to meet your demands,' he added sternly, noticing the captain's intent to object. 'The warehouse manager will show you where the materials are.'

The lieutenant-colonel stepped aside. Donchenko gave the list to Sergey and said, 'I can't really help you pick things out, I don't know anything about medicine. You can put everything in one place by the gate. I'll go back to the truck and see what Maslovsky is up to.'

Gathering the supplies took a lot of time. The warehouse manager, a lithe fellow with black eyes and brown hair, scoured the piles of boxes for the items on the list. He circled round long lines of shelves and admitted guiltily, 'It all arrived last night, and we just finished unloading two hours ago. I can't remember exactly where we put everything.'

Once he'd finished the work, the manager checked it all one last time, before hurrying to the typists to have the necessary paperwork typed up.

Sergey was ecstatic: they'd gotten almost everything they wanted.

Donchenko appeared. Seeing so many supplies, he shook his head in surprise and remarked, 'Look, how much there is! There'll be no place for everything in the truck!'

The warehouse manager came back with the papers in his hand. 'You can load the truck. And you, Comrade Doctor's Assistant, are wanted by the lieutenant-colonel. He is eager to see you. He is over there near the tables.'

The lieutenant-colonel briefly gave Maltsev a task, saying, 'Help the translators. They can't keep up with the work. In Moscow the curfew is lifted at 6:00 a.m. and you can leave then.'

Donchenko nodded and agreed, 'We can't leave just now. The driver needs a rest, otherwise he might fall asleep at the wheel and we'd take a spill.'

Early in the morning the hospital truck, loaded to the very top, started rolling along the silent Moscow streets. Maslovsky reached the Leningrad road just as the rising sun had begun to peek over the horizon and warm the earth.

The sleepless night ensured Sergey's eyes closed as soon as he hit the mattress. He put it on three large boxes in the body of the truck, lay down and instantly fell asleep. He woke up when the truck stopped on the dirt road.

Donchenko knocked loudly on the back of the cab, and said,

'Maltsev, let's swap! Get in the cab!'

Maslovsky sped up as much as was possible on the dirt road and held a piece of rye bread out to Sergey. Seeing how quickly the military doctor's assistant swallowed the bread, the driver murmured, took three potatoes and half an onion out from under the seat, wrapped in a clean rag.

'Treat yourself, Comrade Sergeant. A nurse gave it to me on the way.'

Feeling his cheeks flush, Maslovsky held the steering wheel with his elbows and began to roll a cigarette. Smoking, he drove in silence for some time and then he began to talk about automobiles. Sergey listened patiently and watched the smoke rings.

Suddenly, the driver stopped mid-sentence and

jabbed Sergey with his elbow, 'Look, Comrade Doctor's Assistant, there is something up ahead on the road. It looks like a black dog. Where could it be from? There are no villages nearby.'

Gazing intently into the distance, Sergey noticed a short dark silhouette on the right side of the road. Suddenly the silhouette disappeared. Maslovsky stopped the truck, jumped out of the cab and gestured Sergey to get out. Donchenko jumped out of the truck and asked the pale driver with annoyance,

'Why have you stopped? What's up?'

The captain was going to scold Maslovsky for the delay, but seeing him put a finger to the lips, abruptly stopped.

'There is someone up ahead, might be an ambush.'

Donchenko's eyes widened, and he fidgeted nervously. Then he whispered to Maslovsky in whisper, 'Have you got any weapons?'

'We have everything,' the driver answered quietly, and took out a submachine gun from the box under the driver's seat.

'There it is again,' Sergey pointed at the dark form on the road.

'Drive slowly,' the captain instructed Maslovsky and jumped on the step, 'I'll tell you when to stop.'

'It has disappeared again,' the driver said shaking his head. 'What the hell?'

After about two hundred metres, the truck stopped.

'Our ghost appeared on the road somewhere here,' Maslovsky said and took the submachine gun off safety.

'Let's go into the forest. Keep intervals of fifteen metres!' Donchenko ordered.

Sergey had only taken a few steps into the thicket of pines when he heard a quiet groan to his left. Near a big raspberry bush a woman, dressed in dark clothes, lay on the moss-covered ground. Near her sat a girl of about five, wrapped in a shawl. Holding the woman's hand tightly, the child looked at the approaching man with eyes wide with fright.

Sergey sat down nearby and felt the pulse of the woman's carotid artery. It was weak and slow.

'Wet clothes, cyanosed face; perhaps she has got hypothermia,' he concluded. Sergey quickly headed for the truck.

Maslovsky was standing near the truck holding the start crank. Seeing Sergey, he waved his hand, 'There's nobody in the forest. It was a mirage, or maybe a bear cub that has lost its mother, or some other beast. Get into the cab, Comrade Doctor's Assistant. Soon the captain will be back, he's answering the call of nature in the woods.'

Ignoring the driver, Sergey got into the back of the truck, and took out his greatcoat and the medical kit.

'Where are you going?' Maslovsky asked in surprise.

'There's an unconscious person in the forest,' Sergey answered, quickening his steps.

The woman was lying in the same position. Her eyes were closed, and she was not moving. The child was crying and pulling at the sleeve of the woman's soggy dress.

'Don't worry, we'll bring her around soon,' Sergey said, more to himself than to the child.

Spreading the military coat nearby, he began to take off the woman's clothes, wet and muddy. There was no hint of femininity on her emaciated body.

'Just skin and bones!' gasped Maslovsky as he joined them, 'What happened?'

'Take her clothes,' Sergey ordered with a frown, 'and take the child too.'

He carried the waif-like woman, wrapped in the greatcoat, to the truck. He treaded carefully. The logistics assistant met them coldly, 'All was going well, but hell… how will we take them with us, Comrade Doctor's Assistant?'

'The woman must be put on the mattress, she is suffering from hypothermia and exhaustion,' Sergey answered gloomily. 'We must get her to come to. The child can sit in the cab.'

Maslovsky winked imperceptibly at Sergey and said, 'They should be taken to the hospital, Comrade Captain. The woman has no documents. I searched her clothes. Let the authorities clear up who she is and what she is doing in the front area.'

After thinking for a while, Donchenko announced decisively, 'We'll take her back with us. The commanders can decide then.'

Sergey and the driver put the woman on the mattress. The truck started.

The woman came to with the help of some ammonium chloride. She opened her eyes and looked around blankly, fixing her gaze on the man sitting next to her. Then she asked quietly, almost in a whisper, 'Where am I?'

'We are Soviet military,' Sergey answered quietly. 'We are going to the hospital. I am a doctor.'

'And where is Zinka? Where is my daughter?'

'Don't worry, she is in the cab of the truck.'

Sergey put the medical kit under the woman's ankles and began to rub her feet and wrists. Suddenly remembering something, he knocked on the cab. The truck slowed down and stopped. Maslovsky ran up to the back and asked, 'What's up?'

'Have you got anything to eat?' Sergey asked, looking hopefully at the driver. The driver nodded, ran to the cab, and returned with a rye bread crust. Bending over the tailgate, Sergey broke the bread and held one half out to Maslovsky, saying, 'We must feed the girl. How is she?'

'Fine. We wrapped her in my greatcoat and took off her clothes. She was wet to the waist.'

Sergey broke apart the bread piece by piece and fed the woman. She greedily swallowed the last piece and asked, 'Where are my clothes?'

'They are wet and dirty. Once we reach our destination, you'll be given something to put on. What were you doing alone in the forest with a child? What's your name?'

'Maria.'

The woman sighed as though she feared the doctor wouldn't be interested in her answer and began to tell her story. 'The Germans came to Vasilyevka, our village, a year ago at the beginning of autumn. They built fortifications. All the villagers were evicted from their homes, and we were forced to live in sheds and cow barns. The Germans were very cruel. They beat people for nothing. Very often they raped the young women and girls. And when in winter the Germans were surrounded in a pocket, they slaughtered all our cattle and hens. We were starving then. In summer the Germans withdrew, and the Danes came.'

'Who came?' Sergey asked impatiently.

'Nazi soldiers from Denmark. Many of them were killed when the fighting for Vasilyevka began. It was horrible! Every day bombs and shells were exploding. No house, no shed remained untouched. Everything burned. In spring, my father-in-law built a cellar under the shed, so we hid there. And when the fighting stopped, he said, "Go to east and try to reach the non-occupied zone. Don't walk along the roads, because there are fascists there. Go straight via Neviy Mokh (the name of the bog), save Zinka and yourself." So we set out. I walked in front and Zinka followed me. She got tired quickly, so then I carried her. The day before yesterday I stumbled and got into a quagmire. My bundle was sucked in, but God helped me get out.'

'How many days did you walk?'

'Five.'

Sergey remembered the tea and brought it to her. The woman began to swallow it greedily, holding the greatcoat closed with her other hand. After a few sips, she said suddenly, 'Zinka would like a drink too.'

Craning to see past the piles of supplies into the cab, Sergey said, 'Don't worry, your daughter is asleep on the captain's lap. No sense waking her up, we'll arrive soon.'

The truck trundled along the final stretch of the

route, often sliding and fishtailing from one rut to the next.

The woman's sunken eyes to seem to make up half her face.

'And what will you do with us after we get to the field hospital?' she wondered.

'You'll be treated there. They'll make you feel right at home.'

Sergey suddenly remembered a saying, 'East or West, home is best.'

'They also say there is no place like home,' Maria responded with a shy smile. Looking at Sergey with her big grey eyes, she said something else, but he couldn't make out her words because of the growl of the truck's engine and because his thoughts wandered to private matters.

What he had experienced in the past week – the night raid in No Man's Land, the struggle against spotted fever, the artillery bombardment, the German tank attack, being wounded – all transformed into the image of the blue-eyed girl with a shock of fair hair peeking out from under her field cap, her belt tied tightly around the waist of her uniform's tunic.

'When we arrive, I'll ask to be sent back to the battalion,' Sergey thought resolutely.

In the village, the truck was instantly surrounded by the whole hospital staff. Sokolov looked at the packing slip and embraced in turn the three brave men who had delivered the valuable cargo. He announced to Sergey, his voice brimming with pleasure, 'You are hereby appointed to the position of surgeon. The Army Headquarters' order came this morning. Have a rest after your journey and get ready to work. We have a lot to do.'

'So much for my return to the battalion! This new order is quite the roadblock,' Sergey thought to himself in confusion.

'What's wrong? Aren't you glad?' the head of the hospital looked at Sergey in surprise.

'I'm glad,' said Sergey. 'Yes, I'm glad, Comrade Doctor.'

Sokolov turned to the logistics assistant.

'Begin unloading right away. First, the tents. We'll put them up over there,' the head of the hospital pointed to the edge of the surrounding pine forest. 'We must put some of the wounded there. They will stay there until the cold comes.'

'We picked up a woman with a child on the way back. She was unconscious. She in the cab together with the child. Maltsev gave her first aid,' Captain Donchenko reported.

Sokolov shot a questioning look at Sergey. After he had listened to Maltsev's explanation, he communicated his decision: 'We'll look into the situation. Let her sit there with her child for a while. The lightly wounded soldiers in Wards 7 and 8 are at your disposal, Comrade Maltsev. You, I guess, have some practice in putting up tents. As soon as you put up the tents, transfer the wounded there without delay. Set up stoves too. Captain Donchenko will help you.'

Sergey walked along the only village street and looked around. On the front wall of each house, the ward number was painted in white alongside a big red cross.

Fed with mushroom soup by the ever-present nurse Katerina, Tatyana was blissfully happy. Her wounded back did not ache so much anymore. Lying on one side, she looked through the gap in the curtain at the hospital chief and senior surgeon as they leaned over the table in excitement.

'There are ten packs of ether, each contains one gallon.'

'One gallon?' Sokolov muttered as he poked at a sheet of paper from Moscow. 'Those Yankees! They can't part with miles and pints! How many litres are there?'

'Thirty-nine altogether, Boris Aleksandrovich. And everything necessary for operations and treatment was also received: novocaine, rivanol, phenacetine iodine, codeine, streptocide, glucose, syringes, needles, suturing thread, and five sets of medical instruments.'

'We'll be able to provide for about five hundred wounded men.' The head of the hospital stood up and moved to pick up the telephone receiver. 'I'll try to get blood and solution from Army Medical Command, and you, Gennady, Matveevich, go to Donchenko. Take everything you need and make your rounds. In an hour I'll join you. Tell the captain to find a place for the women in Ward 8.

The head surgeon took the precious invoice and hurried out. On his way, he suddenly remembered something and drew aside Tanya's curtain. Then he said, 'Get ready, my dear, to move to separate "apartments." There you'll be in good company – a refugee woman with a child. So you won't feel lonely.'

Two tight-lipped nurses brought Tanya to the house by stretcher. A woman and a girl of about seven were sitting on the bed near the entrance. Licking their spoons, both of them were heartily eating something from mess tins. The clean floor filled the house with the particular smell of freshly washed wood.

Sergey walked to headquarters as quickly as his half-healed wound permitted. He was going to report to the head of the hospital about moving the lightly wounded soldiers to the tents, which had been put up on the edge of the forest.

In the sky a droning was audible on the horizon, and soon an airplane appeared from among the clouds.

'Rama,' Sergey correctly identified the machine, when he saw the boxy silhouette of the German reconnaissance plane.9

The door of the headquarters opened wide, and Sokolov ran out onto the porch. He looked up and instantly disappeared back into the house. Sergey followed the head of the hospital and saw him shouting at the top of his voice to the telephone receiver:

'Immediately, I beg you! It must be destroyed! We have many badly wounded men. We'll never manage to evacuate them…'

Sokolov replaced the receiver and pronounced gloomily, 'There's no connection.' After a pause he added, 'Nearby there is a regiment of night bombers, but they aren't built to deal with the "Rama." The air regiment commander promised to find a way out. He said he would

---

9   *"Rama," meaning frame in Russian, was the Soviet nickname for the German Focke-Wulf Fw 189 aircraft due to its shape.*

fly himself in a pinch. How are things? Have you pitched the tents?'

Sergey reported on the work done. The head of the hospital nodded and said, 'Slavinsky, the senior surgeon, has just begun his rounds. Find him, he'll tell you what to do next.'

Sergey found the senior surgeon in the house with a red cross and a fat white "2" on the door. Slavinsky was observing a nurse changing the bandage of a soldier wounded in the thigh.

As she lifted the bandage, the nurse let slip a gasp. Little white maggots were squirming around on the wound's surface. The senior surgeon asked Sergey, 'Your thoughts, colleague?'

'Meat fly larvae. They feed on dead tissue: that is why the wound is clean, there is no suppuration.'

'Excellent!' Slavinsky looked at Sergey with interest. 'And what is to be done?'

'The larvae have done what they can. They must be removed. And the wound must be rubbed with Vaseline, and a new bandage applied.'

'And disinfection?'

'It's not necessary. The larvae secretions are bactericidal.'

The surgeon led Sergey to the exit with a pleased smile. He informed Sergey, 'Now we are walking to Number 4, where there is a serious case. He has a shrapnel wound in the forearm with an injured bone. It's a gas gangrene wound, but the infection hasn't gone above the elbow yet. I'll operate on this case today – you and I will operate, to be precise.'

The doctors left the house.

'It's hanging above our heads, like the sword of Damocles,' Sergey said ruefully and pointed at the German plane slowly flying among the white clouds.

'Dear God, that's a...' Slavinsky exclaimed and clasped his hands. 'Does the boss know about it?'

'Yes, he does. He phoned aviation command. They promised to help.'

'But where are they? The "Rama" won't circle for long. It'll fly away soon. Then there'll be a bombing raid.'

It seemed as though the German pilot heard the surgeon's words, as the Focke-Wulf accelerated and climbed away to the west. But at that moment the fading noise of its engines was disturbed by the hum of another motor. A plane with a barrel-shaped fuselage, with red stars on its stubby wings, flew out of the crimson sunset towards the invader.

'That one's ours!' Slavinsky shouted and, momentarily forgetting about the protocol of rank, grabbed his colleague and shook him with excitement.

'It's ours, ours, it's an I-16 "Ishak"!'[10]

Sergey shared the senior surgeon's delight. Raising their heads, the doctors began to watch the dogfight. The I-16 attacked the "Rama" from underneath. Raising its nose, it approached the German plane and began to fire.

'He hit it!' Sergey yelled and clapped his hands.

The I-16 had hit the fuselage of the "Rama" and disabled its right engine. Nevertheless, the German plane kept on flying.

'Damn it! He's still flying on one engine!' Slavinsky cursed as he clenched his fists angrily.

---

10   *Soviet fighter aircraft, Polikarpov I-16, nicknamed "Ishak" (donkey).*

Circling around, the "Rama" dove and began to fire back. The I-16 pilot maneuvered higher, until he in turn dove at his opponent.

The doctors didn't see the end of the dogfight. Both planes quickly flew to the west and disappeared behind the crimson-framed forest horizon.

In the house full of wounded soldiers, Slavinsky quickly walked up to a bed near the window and threw the blanket aside. In answer to the pleading look of the wounded man, an older soldier, he said sharply, 'We have to amputate immediately! Otherwise you'll kick the bucket.'

Gas gangrene painted the left arm of the soldier nearly to the shoulder in an ominous black-blue. Sergey pressed the edge of the wound, which caused a slight crunching sound.

'Crepitation,' Slavinsky said gloomily. 'We must be quick.'

The stretcher-bearers carried the wounded man to the house marked "Operating Theatre." Actually, the operating area, three tables and a wardrobe curtained off, occupied half of the room. The second half was equipped for the medical staff to prepare themselves for surgery.

The doctors began to wash their hands with ammonia solution. Looking at Sergey, Slavinsky asked, 'Have you amputated before?'

'Two times, upper limbs.'

'Where?'

'In the dugout of the battalion medical station.'

The senior surgeon's hands stopped moving, and there was surprise on his face. He remarked, 'Battalion doctor's assistants are not provided with surgical instruments. They have no right to perform operations. Why didn't you evacuate the wounded to the regimental medical point?'

'The battalion had been encircled by the enemy for three days. Amputations were necessary for the patients to survive. Gas gangrene.'

The senior surgeon began to wipe his hands bitterly.

'This will be a guillotine amputation,' he resolutely said to Sergey and the nurse, a plump, dark-haired woman of middle age, after all preparations had been completed.

The stretcher-bearers put the soldier, stripped to the waist, on the operating table. They strapped the soldier's arm on a small table they placed next to it. The nurse put a gauze bandage on the soldier's face. The sharp smell of ether filled the air. Sergey, standing at the head of the bed, watched the patient's eyes carefully. The movement of the eyes gradually stopped in the centre. Sergey held his palms down over the eyes. Then he quickly jerked them away. The pupils didn't react to the light of the reflective lamp.

The nurse felt the soldier's pulse and gave the all clear sign with her eyes. Sergey did the same after catching the glance of the surgeon. Slavinsky nodded. He selected an amputating scalpel with his gloved hand. He closed his eyes for a second, opened them and quickly walked to the soldier lying on the operation table.

Sergey assisted with great interest. He had helped the wounded at the front for fourteen months – in bomb and shell craters, in ditches and holes, and even in out in the open. He had hidden them from the enemy bullets behind tree trunks, or occasional boulders. Sometimes he had been completely helpless, because in his field kit there were no surgical instruments like those now in the expert hands of the senior surgeon.

After finishing the operation, the doctors went out onto the porch and, sitting on the steps, they breathed in the fragrant forest.

'You assisted well, I've no complaints,' Slavinsky said approvingly. 'And you put in the ligatures quickly and skillfully. The next operation you will do yourself. Today we have two more. In Ward 2 there is…'

The surgeon didn't finish his thought: the head of the hospital suddenly appeared from around the corner of the house.

'Sit down, sit down,' he waved his hand to the doctors, who had begun to stand up. He sat down on the well-worn step. Then he took out a cigarette with a trembling hand from the cigarette-case, lit it and greedily inhaled the smoke.

'What happened, Boris Aleksandrovich?' the head surgeon asked, anxiously looking at the troubled face of the hospital chief.

'The air regiment headquarters phoned. That "Rama," which had been circling over the hospital, was destroyed over our front line. The German pilot didn't manage to get to the Nazi lines.

'That's great, isn't it?!' Slavinsky burst out gladly. 'The I-16 pilot saved the hospital from being bombed. He is a real hero!'

Sokolov flicked the ash to the ground, finished the cigarette, opened the cigarette-case again and said quietly, 'The commander of the air regiment may be awarded the "Hero of the Soviet Union" posthumously. He rammed the enemy plane and went down as well.'

Without taking a new cigarette, the head of the hospital snapped his cigarette case shut and commanded, 'Everyone follow me to headquarters. We'll have dinner and pray for the pilot.'

In the headquarters, as soon as the doctors sat down at the table, the telephone rang. Sokolov listened to the voice on the line, saying from time to time: 'yes', 'it's clear', 'we'll get ready.' When the conversation was over, he put the bottle of spirits back in the safe and turned to his subordinate.

'The Army Medical Command has announced a state of combat readiness number one. This means that our offensive will start in the morning. Our task is to examine the wounded immediately and determine those who are to be evacuated to the rear hospital. The first six wards, Gennady Matveevich, are yours. 7 to 12 are mine. Maltsev will examine the patients in the tents. In an hour and a half, we'll meet here in the headquarters again. I want to hear your suggestions on gathering the wounded men. We have so much to do that the staff will hardly have time to sleep tonight.'

Looking at Sergey, he added, 'The surgeon and I are used to this. "Readiness Number One" has now been announced to us, let God remember, for the sixth time. It happens before each offensive. This is the current situation, Comrade Doctor.'

Surprised at being addressed with a rank above his own, Sergey looked at the head of the hospital with surprise. Had he misheard?

'I was going to tell you at morning roll call, but the situation has changed, and there's no time for festivities now.' Sokolov handed collar patches with three cubes on a dark-green background to Sergey.

'Congratulations! The order to commission you as an officer arrived this morning.'

He quickly shook the hand of the new army doctor and hurried to the exit.

The senior surgeon said a few parting words to Sergey on the steps of the porch: 'When examining the men, make up a list of all those requiring surgery. And drop in on ward number 4 and see how our women are getting on.'

Sergey saw the forest refugees on the bench near the fence, in the front garden of house number 4. Maria wore a black dress and a sleeveless jacket, and was helping her daughter make a toy from sticks and branches.

'Why aren't you in the ward?' Sergey admonished the mother. Then he looked at the girl, who had stopped building in fright.

'We've come here to play and sit in the sun. She is bored in the house, so she makes noise, and the wounded girl in there needs a rest.'

Having arranged the child's hair, Maria arranged her own, looked at the doctor and gave him a beautiful smile.

'I have to examine you and your daughter, so you'll

have to stop playing. I'll be waiting for you in the ward.'

In the house, on the bed near the window, a fair-haired young woman with a wound in her back was sleeping. Her hand hung down from the bed, almost touching the floor.

'Her breathing is regular,' Sergey thought mechanically and placed the stool at the head of the bed. He sat down and reached towards the patient's carotid artery to check the pulse. His arm froze halfway. Blood rushed to Sergey's head: his patient was Tanya, first company medical instructor, the girl he had thought about constantly since he'd seen her for the first time.

Sergey took Tanya's hand, put it on his knees and began to gently stroke her thin white palm and delicate fingers.

He did not see Maria and Zinka enter the house. He did not see how they stood staring at the doctor caressing the hand of the wounded girl in their ward.

THE TRAIN OF HOPE

The dust rose over the narrow dirt road, raised by horses' hooves and creaking cart wheels. Sometimes, a gust of hot June wind scattered a long dusty cloud and drove it away over the field, where ears of winter wheat were maturing. But when the wind died away, that thick dusty veil, dimming the afternoon sunlight, rose again over the road.

The dust lay in a thick coat on the face, neck, and collar of the military man who walked alongside the lead cart. So much of it covered his tunic that that one could hardly make out the emblem in the form of a snake's head and ceremonial cup.

The man was falling asleep as he moved. With a tired look in his sleepy eyes he threw a cursory glance at the broad back of the driver, or at the Red Army men lying in the cart, or at the sickly shrubs along the road. Sometimes the soldier stumbled, and, so as not to fall down, grabbed onto the side of the cart.

The man was overtaken by a fair-haired girl in a drab-coloured uniform. She saluted, took a sheet of paper from her breast pocket, gave it a look, and began to speak. In her other hand, she held a bag with a red cross on it. The girl must have told the man something very important, because he suddenly stopped, and, massaging his temples with one hand, asked with annoyance, 'How many? Repeat please!'

'Nine, Comrade Doctor,' the girl answered in a loud voice and stopped, slowly lowering the sheet of paper.

'We won't even carry half of the wounded,' the man said angrily. Looking at the girl, he ordered in a hoarse voice, 'Run to the end of the column, find Tarasenko and tell him not to tarry. Tell him to take care of the lightly wounded soldiers. Those lagging behind should be given seats in the carts. We must move much faster.'

Sending the girl off, the doctor caught up with the lead cart and shouted to the driver, 'Come on! Let's go faster!'

He sat down on the driving box and asked, 'Can we get to Baranovichy in an hour?'

The coachman obliged, with the cry of 'Gee up, faster, you damned nag!' He answered the question leisurely, stretching out his words, 'Why not? God willing, we'll get there. Behind that wood there is the town.'

The driver cracked the whip towards the forest. A short man in civilian clothes ran up on the cart. Panting heavily, he reported to the doctor, 'Nine soldiers have died, Comrade Vetkin: blood loss, shock, internal bleeding. Two lightly wounded soldiers have lost consciousness. There is no water and our bandages are running out, there's no ammonium chloride…'

'I know, I know everything, Aleksander Iosifovich,' the doctor stopped him angrily and jumped off the cart. 'We must be patient. It is five kilometres to go to Baranovichy, not more. I hope to get help in the town. The main thing for us now is to reach the forest as soon as possible. There we will be less noticeable to the German aircraft.

Twenty minutes later, about thirty carts laden with wounded soldiers lying "head to tail," the medical truck (drawn by two horses as there was no fuel), and a disorderly crowd of walking wounded plunged into the cool sanctuary of the forest.

'Halt! Fifteen minutes!' Vetkin announced, shaking the dust from his sleeves.

'Halt, halt' the command spread along the column of carts.

Looking for the fair hair of the senior nurse, the doctor walked to the end of the column. He found her near a cart with badly wounded men. Bending over a groaning soldier, the nurse carefully wiped the sweat from his thin face.

Vetkin came up nearer and saw the soldier, whom they had found on the bank of the river Shchara in the morning. The shrapnel wound on his shin had turned gangrenous, and the deadly infection was mercilessly eating away his flesh. But neither the doctor nor the rest of the medical staff could help him.

'Distribute all emergency rations to the nurses and medics,' said the doctor, nodding at the nurse's medical bag. 'Then change the bandages.' Then he asked,

'Are there any spirits left?'

'In the bottom of the tin, less than fifty millilitres.'

'Give it to him,' Vetkin instructed.

First Sergeant Tarasenko, looking anxious, jogged up to the cart. Wiggling his wheat-hued moustache, he blurted out, 'The lightly wounded have kicked up a fuss; you are wanted, Comrade Doctor.'

Frowning, Vetkin walked to the tail of the column.

Once the team was given the order to halt, some of the lightly wounded walked over to the bushes. Some sat dawn on the ground and leaned on the trunks of the roadside trees. They kept silent and closed their eyes in an attempt to absorb some strength from the forest air after the long march.

A group of about a dozen men were discussing something in a small clearing near the road. One of them, with a bandaged arm, rushed to the doctor as he approached.

'Come have a look at this, Comrade Doctor,' drawled the soldier, opening wide his gap-toothed mouth and waving with his healthy arm.

'You consider all of us lightly wounded, but five of our fellows can't even walk, and we are dragging them along by the arms.'

'You shouldn't shout, Comrade Soldier' Vetkin said, his voice betraying his exhaustion. 'We'll soon settle everything. Take them out to the clearing.'

Quickly examining the five soldiers, the doctor declared to the men around him, 'You're right. They can't walk. We'll find place for them in the carts.'

'In every cart there are four wounded men. What are we going to do, stack them up?' a voice said from the crowd.

'We'll find a place for them,' Vetkin said curtly.

Near the column's very last cart, he saw Tarasenko

and caught his attention, calling, 'Walk along the column. The drivers are all old village hands, they must have brought some shovels for the trip. We need about eight.'.

Everyone helped dig the grave in the forest glade, including the drivers and the medical staff. The fourteen dead were saluted three times from the barrel of Vetkin and Tarasenko's service pistols. The badly wounded soldiers were then placed on the carts in the places freed by the dead. The column kept on moving.

At the edge of the forest, the lead cart was stopped by a sharp shout: 'Halt! The leader of the group come out!'

From behind a thick spruce, a tall soldier with a machine gun at the ready and binoculars around his neck walked out onto the road. Having determined Vetkin's role and rank, the man raised his hand to his blue-banded cap and said crisply, 'Senior Lieutenant of the People's Commissariat for Internal Affairs Lutsenko. This is a checkpoint. Show your documents, Comrade Doctor.'

The soldier returned the ID to Vetkin and raised his hand. Out from behind the trees about ten soldiers emerged, clad in new uniforms with blue collar patches. At a signal from their commander, they divided into two groups and moved down each side of the road, weapons at the ready.

The senior lieutenant told Vetkin to step aside, and asked him quietly, 'Where have you come from?'

'From Slonim,' the doctor answered impatiently. 'The medical battalion of the 169th Infantry Division, or what remains of it.' Looking into the eyes of the senior lieutenant, he added forcefully, 'I have more than two hundred wounded men with me, and many of them need urgent treatment.'

'I won't keep you long. I see my soldiers coming back already. Have you noticed any suspicious people in your group?'

Vetkin shook his head negatively.

'Where are the cart drivers from?' the officer went on asking.

'From Tomilino,' the doctor answered sharply, beginning to get angry. 'Animal-drawn transport has been mobilized there. As soon as they bring the wounded to the town, they will go back home.'

One of the soldiers ran up said something into the senior lieutenant's ear.

The officer nodded. Addressing Vetkin, he said, 'You may continue, Comrade Doctor. It is three kilometres from here to the station. Address the commandant for any problems. In the town there is…'

He suddenly stopped talking in mid-sentence and looked up at the sky. Vetkin had also heard the growing drone of aircraft engines. Raising his head, the army doctor tried to see the approaching airplanes in the sky, but the high spruces and birches hung over the forest road. Through this green forest tunnel, the sky appeared as little more than a narrow blue strip.

'Germans,' said the senior lieutenant, who had darted out to get a better look. Then, his face darkening, he spat, 'They're going to bomb the town again, the monsters!'

Taking deep breath, he shouted with all his might, 'Air

raid! Nobody move! Don't leave the forest! No smoking!'

The dull boom of explosions, the shrieking of the German dive-bombers, and frequent barking of machine guns indicated to those in the forest that the nearby town was locked in an unequal struggle against an enemy who had dropped from the clouds.

The senior lieutenant chose a thick birch on the forest edge, climbed it and, sitting on a branch, began to share what he saw.

'There are six of them, the vultures,' he called down to Vetkin and the others. 'It looks like they are flying towards the station.'

In the din, the sounds of the planes, bombs and machine guns could no longer be told apart.

'It's burning,' the senior lieutenant furiously cried, throwing his arms in the air and nearly losing his balance. 'It's burning, the dirty swine! Aha! They've got one!'

Leaning down, he gladly reported, 'On the roof of the station there are four antiaircraft machine guns. Great job, gunners!'

The explosions and gunfire then subsided as suddenly as it had begun.

The senior lieutenant of the People's Commissariat for Internal Affairs (NKVD) climbed down from the birch tree, and the carters who had hidden in the heart of the forest climbed atop their carts again.

Vetkin gave the command, "Forward!" and jumped onto the lead cart. The column left the forest and made its way to the town, which was veiled in smoke and flame.

The station master was glad to see the doctor. Pouring

strong tea into a thin glass in a metal holder, he spoke in a muted baritone, 'Yesterday, we received a telegramme from the People's Commissariat of Communication. It was an order to arrange medical trains to evacuate wounded soldiers and officers to the rear. So you have come in time.'

He opened a drawer, took out two sheets of paper with the telegraph text, and handed them to Vetkin.

'Here you are, Comrade Doctor, the full text.'

The telephone rang. The station master began to shout something into the receiver. He leaned away from the doctor and spoke in a lower tone. Vetkin sipped the strong, sweet tea and began reading. The telegramme of the People's Commissariat gave instructions and dates for arranging the hospital trains, the number and type of carriages, train crew and much else besides. It emphasized that the main task of the military trains was to quickly evacuate the wounded men to the rear.

A man in uniform military man with three cubes on his collar entered the office where Vetkin and the railway station master were sitting. He saluted the doctor and introduced himself.

'I'm the station commandant, Senior Lieutenant Kalinich.' He looked out the window and asked, 'Are those your wounded soldiers, Comrade Doctor?'

Vetkin nodded and responded enthusiastically, 'They all need to be put somewhere, especially those who are seriously injured. Some of them need urgent treatment. I have no medicine, I have nothing. We must give them food and drink. They haven't eaten anything for two days.'

'The accommodation is ready, it's over there on track number three,' the commandant pointed out the window. Fourteen carriages. Two are set up for the seriously injured. The rest of carriages have been prepared for the medical staff, for the train crew, for a kitchen, for a first aid station. We've equipped carriages for cooking, for bandaging, washing, and storing food. Everything has been done according to the instructions of Communications Command.'

'In that case I will begin loading the wounded,' Vetkin said and started for the door.

'There is no bedding or mattresses on the train. Other things are also

needed,' the commandant said, stopping him. 'You can get everything you need from the city warehouses. There are still fires burning in that part of town, I'm not sure what's going on there.'

'Nevertheless, they must be put in the carriages right away, we have to get them out of the baking sun,' Vetkin insisted. 'I'll go to the warehouses right away. But we have no petrol in our ambulance. Not a drop. Can you help us?'

The commandant nodded. He took out a clean sheet of paper.

'I'm going to write a note to the town commandant. I'm sure he is in the area of the fires. He can approve everything you need. Go there immediately, and I will start getting your wounded where they belong.'

'Nurse Sosnovskaya, Master Sergeant Tarasenko, and Doctor Greenberg will help you,' Vetkin said, and looked out the window, trying to find the surgeon's stout figure amongst the walking wounded.

While the commandant was busy looking for fuel, Vetkin quickly went through all the carriages and examined the equipment of the ambulance train. In three carriages, the compartment partitions had been partially removed. This allowed them to be used for storing food, water, drugs, and bandages, and to convert others into rooms for bandaging, washing, cooking. In one of the carriages all the partitions had been removed, leaving only a small table in the middle.

'Probably for the staff,' Vetkin thought, remembering what was written in the telegram.

Filled with fuel, the ambulance truck rolled along the streets towards the black smoke in the town centre, which hung like the train of a funeral dress in the cloudless summer sky.

The commandant's face was darkened with soot and devoid of emotion. Glancing at the paper he was shown, he hurriedly wrote some additional words and, waving his hand towards the concrete fence, ran off to a nearby fire-engine which had pulled up to a burning building.

The warehouses were behind the fence. Military and civilians were scurrying about, busy loading various barrels, bundles, and boxes onto the trucks and carts parked at the gate.

'Medicine and medical equipment are in storehouse number six, food is in number two, and mattresses, blankets, pillows and underwear are in warehouse ten,' said a breathless man in a dark blue overall, dirty with oil and flour. 'You will load yourselves, because I haven't got anybody for that. See what's going on around here?' he nodded towards the burning building. 'If the bombs had hit fifty metres to the right, the storehouses – and we – would be nothing but a memory.'

'We'll load by ourselves,' Vetkin hurriedly agreed. He jumped into the cab and told the driver, 'Full speed to warehouse six!'

It took the doctor and the driver half an hour to load the ambulance to the top with food and medical equipment.

'You're a little tired, aren't you?' Vetkin remarke,d and winked at the driver.

'No, not at all, Comrade Doctor.' the soldier responded. He smiled and deftly turned the wheel, navigating along the streets packed with trucks, carts, and refugees moving east.

The platform and the station were also crowded with people escaping the war. Senior Lieutenant Kalinich was running and shouting alongside a line of soldiers. He was trying to show his organizing skills in packing the refugees into freight carriages.

In the station master's office, veiled with smoke, the telephone rang all the time, and uniformed railway men scurried hither and thither. They were signing papers, demanding something, arguing and debating. In the corner, an NKVD officer put his notepad on his knee and scribbled something down with his pencil.

Noticing Vetkin, the officer put the pad away and declared loudly, 'Your wounded soldiers have already been put on the train. The ambulance train must depart immediately, Comrade Doctor.'

'I've gotten the medicine and some of the food so far,' Vetkin answered frowning. 'We still need mattresses, bedding, kitchen equipment, and many other things. All that means two or three trips with the ambulance.'

The NKVD captain adjusted his cap and led the doctor to a corner of the room. He then said quietly, 'Our troops didn't manage to break out of the encirclement on the river Shchara. The Germans are near Slonim now. In a few hours, I think, they will reach Baranovichy. There might be more air raids. Make haste.'

'What about the carts? Have you sent them back?' Vetkin asked anxiously.

'Of course not. They're behind the station. I ordered two soldiers to watch over your carts and drivers.'

'Can I take them as guards?'

The officer nodded and began to mark something on his pad again. Looking thankfully at the captain, the doctor hurried away.

In the storehouses, Vetkin loaded the carts and the ambulance with mattresses and bedding.

'You've cleaned us right out, Comrade Doctor,' the storehouse manager said with a smile and closed the gate of the building with a long bolt. 'Two hundred eighty-two sets of bedding.'

'That's enough, even a little extra,' Vetkin thought with satisfaction, climbed into the ambulance and gave an order to the carters, who were sitting on their carts, 'Follow me, single file.'

The engine coughed and the truck moved, slowly leaving the warehouse area into the street. The horse-drawn carts soon fell in line behind it.

At the crossing, the column's path was suddenly blocked by a cyclist, an elderly man in a white doctor's smock over a pair of pants. He explained, 'I'm the head physician at the town hospital. The railway station commandant telephoned me and said you're in charge of the hospital train. The ground floor of the hospital is packed with your wounded soldiers.'

'What do you mean "my" wounded soldiers?' Vetkin responded in surprise.

'I mean soldiers, other ranks and officers. The day before yesterday they were brought here, almost as soon as it all started. I think—'

'How many are there?'

'There are sixty left. Two died yesterday, one died before that. You know, colleague, we—'

Vetkin again interrupted the man, 'Is there any transport at the hospital?'

'We've got two medical vans.'

'How many badly wounded are there?'

'Only eleven. Three amputated legs, two pneumothorax cases, four craniocerebral wounds.'

'Understood,' Vetkin interrupted the hospital doctor one more time.

'Load all the badly wounded and go to the station right away. Our train has red crosses painted on the carriages. We leave in an hour from now, not later. I suppose your van is designed to carry four bed cases and two sitting cases. There are two medical vans, GAZ-55 model trucks.'

'Right,' the hospital doctor nodded. 'Two wounded soldiers on suspended stretchers and five on turn-down seats. We'll evacuate all of them in four trips.'

'Who has been caring for your patients?' Vetkin asked, looking at his watch.

'Our medical staff. Most of the wounded men came in a freight carriage. They were accompanied by a military medical assistant. He is with them now, at the hospital.'

'Well, Comrade...I don't know your name,' Vetkin began, looking at the dark-haired doctor with a receding hairline.

'Aleksander Iosifovich,' the man answered quickly, and turned his head to hear the army doctor better.

'Aleksander Iosifovich, please bring all the wounded to the train. Again, you have only one hour.'

'Understood,' the dark-haired doctor said crisply. He hesitated an instant and asked in a strained voice, 'Can we put civilian patients from our hospital onto the hospital train?'

Vetkin was about to answer a sharp 'No! 'Military personnel only,' but, seeing the despair etched on the man's face, changed his mind.

'How many patients do you have?'

'About fifteen. I can put a doctor and a nurse at your disposal to accompany them.

'Agreed,' Vetkin said and got into the ambulance and waved to the doctor.

The loaded column headed for the station. A freight

train departed from the station and quickly gathered speed. The locomotive, sending clouds of black smoke into the sky, pulled about twenty freight carriages. All of them were packed with people escaping the disaster.

At the entrance to the station, Vetkin ran into the NKVD captain. He was carrying two big suitcases. Four soldiers followed him. They were pulling a big object wrapped in canvas. The officer set the suitcases down on the concrete floor and caught his breath. Looking at the doctor, he announced: 'If you don't leave in half an hour, you and your wounded men will end up be in enemy hands. The Germans have broken through our lines near Slonim.

The captain snatched up his suitcases and went onto the platform, followed by his men. Vetkin rushed to the square near the station.

'Unload and be quick!' he shouted loudly to the carters. 'Follow me to the green carriages with the red crosses! Get a move on!'

Emphasizing the importance of the moment, Vetkin took his pistol out of the holster and shot two times into the air. The cart drivers sprang into action. Some of the lightly wounded soldiers helped them to unload the carts. Soon all the equipment had been put on the train.

'Thank you for the help! You can go home!' the doctor shouted and waved good-bye to the owners of the carts.

Whipping their horses, the peasants hurried back to Tomilino. Vetkin ran to the station master. He had to get in touch with the rear to inform them about the loss of the divisional medical battalion in the bombing, the breakout, the number of wounded, the ambulance train, and to ask for further instructions about the route.

All his intentions, however, soon came to naught: in the station master's office two railway men were hurriedly packing a big box with files of documents, books, stacks of paper, boxes, and stationary.

'Minsk was bombed all day yesterday, we haven't been able to reach them since. No communication at all,' the station master answered Vetkin. Just then he snapped off the telephone wire with a jerk and handed the apparatus to the railway man. 'Put it into the box, we'll need it in the new place.'

Just then, the station commandant rushed in, his tunic wet through with sweat. He announced, 'The freight train has just left, and there are no more working engines. Three are being repaired.'

'What can they possibly repair now?!' the station master said angrily. 'Have them join our carriage to the ambulance train, and go straight to Mogilev.'

'Why Mogilev?' Vetkin asked. 'The Front Headquarters and Medical Services Department are in Minsk. If we get there, they'll define our route, and provide food and supplies for the rest of the journey.'

'Half an hour ago NKVD Captain Korovin said that the authorities had left Minsk at night and headed for Mogilev.'

Embarrassed by the news, Vetkin kept silent.

'There is no help for us in Minsk,' the commandant objected with a frown.

'Now all of us here are officers, Comrade Doctor,' the station master said with a sigh. 'Go, I ask you, to the train. Soon another carriage will be coupled on, and we'll leave at once. I hope there will be no new air raids.'

'Why wouldn't there be?' Vetkin asked in disbelief.

'The Germans are probably about to enter the town and want to seize the station with its staff, equipment, and tracks undamaged. And we, as ill luck would have it, have neither blasting charges nor sappers.'

Near the ambulance train, refugees had crowded the third track. There were a lot of them – old women, young women with babies and older children, men, breadwinners, grey-haired old men, and teenagers. For all of them, as for the wounded on the train, the hospital train was their last hope of salvation from the threat of death approaching from the west.

When the doctor appeared near the lead carriage, the crowd surrounded him, their shouts merging into an unintelligible cacophony. Looking first right, then left, Vetkin saw faces twisted with fear, and anxiety-filled eyes begging for sympathy. He couldn't bring himself to ignore them – he saw in them the same problems and fears that had befallen him these last four days.

A dark-haired refugee pressed her baby, wrapped in a small blanket, to her bosom. With her other hand, she grabbed the doctor's sleeve and cried in a shrill, piercing voice, 'Take us with you! They will kill us!' It seemed to Vetkin as though her entreaty flowed into him straight out of her large black eyes, wide with horror.

Elbowing his way through the crowd, the station

commandant, Kalinich, managed to reach Vetkin.

'The Germans are not far!' he shouted as loudly as he could. 'Do you hear that?'

The crowd suddenly quieted; the hollow thump of artillery fire sounded in the distance.

'Our troops are fighting somewhere west of Anisimovichy,' the commandant said, wiping his wet face with his sleeve.

'Can we couple some more carriages to our train, for the refugees?' Vetkin asked anxiously.

The senior lieutenant shook his head doubtfully.

'I'm not sure; we could ask the driver, but…' lowering his voice to a whisper, he said with a sigh, 'The locomotive crew has run off. We're in a real bind.'

'Where has it run off to?' Vetkin asked in surprise.

'In different directions. Traitors!' he swore. 'It'll be alright,' he continued reassuringly to calm the sweating doctor, 'We'll do our best. Kuvaldin, the station master, will couple our carriage, and he himself will drive the train. I'll help him, and some of the young men and boys from among the refugees will work as stokers.'

'Please, ask him about additional carriages,' Vetkin implored worriedly.

'I'll ask,' the commandant said after looking at the crowd of refugees. 'I think we can fit them all into four roofed freight cars.'

The refugees, who had been listening to the conversation, began to applaud loudly and a few shouted their thanks.

The commandant trotted off to look for Kuvaldin.

Vetkin climbed aboard the lead carriage. A tall thin man sitting near the window, upon seeing the doctor, stood up.

'I'm one of the train crew,' he said quietly. 'I am a driver. My surname is Sokolov.'

Vetkin introduced himself briefly, 'Doctor Vetkin, responsible for this hospital train.' He shook the driver's hand and asked, 'Who else is part of your team?'

'Conductors, the train foreman, and the electrician. The conductors are in the other cars now, they are helping the medical staff. The electrician and the foreman are checking the condition of the carriages.'

Vetkin looked out the window of their compartment and noticed the town hospital ambulances slowly pulling onto the platform. He jumped out of the carriage to meet the new arrivals. As he did so, he addressed the crowd:

'In these trucks there are badly-wounded soldiers. I ask the men among you to help us load them onto the train.'

There were more than enough volunteers, to whom Vetkin gave instructions on the run.

A young red-haired man in a white coat jumped out of the cab of the lead ambulance. Introducing himself as 'Nikolai Khomenko, surgeon', he reported, 'We have brought all the badly wounded, sixteen men. The walking wounded are on their way. Eleven seriously ill patients will come with the second trip.'

Suddenly, Senior Nurse Sosnovskaya appeared. Her coat was spotted with blood. She caught the doctor's eye and burst out, 'All the wounded have been accommodated, Vladimir Ivanovich: mattresses have been set out;

everything has been done. Master Sergeant Tarasenko fed all the wounded – we made sandwiches and tea for them.'

'What's that? Vetkin pointed at the spots on the coat.

'Operation,' the nurse explained, covering the spots with her hands. 'Aleksander Iosifovich amputated Zalozajev's arm, he had gangrene.'

Vetkin was dumbfounded. 'What operation!?' he exclaimed, 'Have you and Greenberg gone crazy! In unhygienic conditions!?'

'Not in unhygienic conditions, Vladimir Ivanovich,' the senior nurse's tone was offended. 'Tarasenko gave us a bottle of spirits and I washed all the instruments. We used it for our hands, masks, and coats. Everything was done according to the rules. Aleksander Iosifovich said that there could be no delay, otherwise it could be too late. And how well he operates! With two hands! I've never seen such skill in my eight years as a nurse.'

'Well, well. The consequences of an operation carried out in such conditions are not yet clear,' Vetkin grumbled. 'Return to him and continue to assist. What made you leave the operating room?'

'Aleksander Iosifovich is treating the wound now. He needs a quarter of an hour to finish. He sent me to find out when we were leaving.'

'Run back to him,' Vetkin ordered, 'and tell him we depart in twenty minutes.'

Turning to the town hospital surgeon, he stated confidently, 'Perhaps at the front such things may be the norm. The great Pirogov, I think, may have had to face such situations himself.' 11

---

11   *N. I. Pirogov (1810-1881), Russian pioneer of field surgery.*

The fair-haired surgeon said to Vetkin, 'There are practically no patients left in the local hospital. I have brought those who are seriously ill. The rest went home, they are afraid of the bombing and what might happen next. The head physician has asked that you include the hospital staff reservists. Many of us received a summons from the military commissariat, but when we came to the enlistment office this morning it was closed.'

'And how many of you were called up?' Vetkin asked briskly.

'Eight: the doctor, the medical assistant, three nurses, and three junior nurses.'

Vetkin sighed with relief. His head had been spinning since the beginning of the hospital train saga, trying to reckon how the head of a bombed out medical station, Dr. Greenberg from Grodno (who joined them near the river Shchara), and Liza Sosnovskaya (the last surviving nurse) were to care for hundreds of wounded.

Vetkin latched onto this solution to his problem as a drowning man to a life ring.

'I'll take those who can be ready in five minutes,' the doctor said, and clapped Khomenko on the shoulder. 'Follow them and be quick. Soon our ambulance will join the others. Just remember: time is running out.'

The station master coupled five freight carriages to the hospital train with a switching engine. The refugees rushed in and filled four of them. The commandant and four men began to maneuver an anti-aircraft machine gun onto the roof of the fifth and last car.

'It'll be safer this way,' the commandant said to Vetkin. 'Knocking out the speedy German planes is quite difficult, but the boys will do their best to prevent any accurate enemy bombardment.'

The senior lieutenant cut the conversation short and began to oversee the raising of the guns.

'Lift the left edge! Again left! Together!' he shouted to the soldiers whose faces were red from the strain. 'The swivel is caught. A bit lower! Be careful! Don't bend the shoulder rests!'

The second ambulance convoy arrived with twenty lightly wounded men. As the first truck arrived at the platform, the town hospital staff spilled out one after the other.

'Almost everyone wanted to go with the medical train,' Khomenko explained, throwing up his hands with a guilty look.

'We'll find something for them to do' Vetkin said, trying to calm him down. 'Where are the rest of the wounded? How many of them are there?'

'Sixteen, Comrade Doctor. There was no place for all of them in the trucks.'

'You should have put them in the trucks. I see your girls are young. They could have come on foot,' Vetkin said in an accusatory tone.

'Here they are,' Khomenko pointed at a group of walking wounded who had just reached the square in front of the station, 'And Medical Assistant Kupriyanov is with them.'

Wiping his hands with a dirty towel, Kuvaldin came up to Vetkin. 'We can go,' he announced, looking at the guns on the roof of the carriage. 'We'll get to Mogilev via Slutsk. It will be some three hundred kilometres. We can drive to Gomel via Kalinkovichy, but that route is a hundred kilometres longer.'

'If only we knew where the Germans are,' the hospital doctor said. 'Let's get moving first, and we'll work out a solution on the way.'

Kuvaldin looked at the station commandant, standing proudly next to the anti-aircraft car and said, 'Come here, Mikhalych, and get into the locomotive. You'll help. And take two soldiers – they will work as stokers.'

As he was about to get into the locomotive, he warned Vetkin, 'I think that on the way we will have to signal to you more than once. Two long whistles – air raid, two short – approaching a station, three long – danger. Trying to go too fast won't work, the train is overloaded, and we might have trouble with the brakes.' Slightly smiling, he confessed, 'I also need some time to get comfortable. I haven't driven a train in ten years.'

The locomotive gave a long whistle and pulled nine-teen carriages full of wounded soldiers and refugees out of the station towards the southeast.

Vetkin stood in the vestibule of the carriage and pon-dered his next steps. His thoughts were scattered after the unbearable stress of the past four days. They flashed across his mind in no discernible order, mixed into one another in a feverish heap.

'Calm down, calm down. You are responsible for three hundred people, you need to focus,' Vetkin commanded to himself. He began to massage his temples; sometimes it helped clear his mind. Then he opened the door with a jerk and resolutely walked into the carriage.

Near one of the windows stood a tall man with gray-ing temples wearing a railway worker's uniform. Seeing the doctor, he stepped towards him and introduced himself: 'Senior Train Conductor Aleksey Dmitriyevich Yerokhin.'

'There's a war on, but his uniform is clean and ironed. The man likes his work,' Vetkin thought, pleased. He shook hands with the conductor and said, 'Aleksey Dmitriyevich, please gather the train crew train and the medical staff in the headquarters carriage.'

The conductor hurried to carry out the order. Walk-ing from carriage to carriage, Vetkin surveyed the neat, clean beds and the patients lying in them with satisfaction. Exhausted, the wounded were all asleep.

The doctors, nurses, and train crew gathered in the carriage. All of them, young and old, civilians and military, looked at the doctor in expectation. Vetkin didn't see fear in their faces, rather one question: 'What are we to do?'

'We are,' he began in an even, confident tone, 'to take the wounded and sick soldiers and the refugees to the safe area where they can be treated properly. Mogilev, where we are now headed, will be the end of the first stage of our journey.'

'And then?' a young grey-eyed nurse asked.

'You are interrupting! Let us listen!' someone hushed her.

'Later we'll get new orders according to military developments,' Vetkin answered calmly. 'I expect you will follow the strictest military discipline.'

He looked at his watch and began to give orders.

'The senior nurse will have to sort out the junior staff for the care of the wounded. The list of nurses appointed to each carriage must be given to me. Doctors Greenberg and Khomenko will examine the badly wounded and treat them immediately. Master Sergeant Tarasenko will prepare supper by five o'clock. Choose helpers from among the lightly wounded. Report to me about the quantity of food available. Any questions?'

'I have a question, Comrade Doctor,' the senior conductor coughed into his fist, raised his pale eyes and asked, 'The station master hasn't informed me about our signals, and the crew must know when to get ready for stops, and all that...'

'Yes, Aleksey Dmitriyevich,' Vetkin agreed, 'thank you for reminding me. Listen everybody! The main signal is three long whistles, which means danger ahead. If that happens, we have to—'

Just then, three long whistle blasts erupted from the locomotive. Everybody rushed to the windows.

'It looks like we're coming up on Kletsk station,' the senior conductor announced, observing the neat wooden houses in well-tended front gardens.

Suddenly his long, thin figure stiffened, then bent double as he cried, 'Get down! The Germans!'

Not many of the staff followed his example. Most of them, leaning on the windows of the carriage, wanted to see with their own eyes those who on Sunday had attacked their Motherland, ruthlessly bringing death and ruin.

On the station platform stood two armed motorcycles. Military men in unknown light grey uniforms were sitting in them and looking attentively at the approaching train. Two of them got off of the motorcycles and came up to the edge of the platform. As the locomotive pulled alongside the Germans, the engine suddenly covered them with a powerful white cloud.

'Way to go, boys!' the train electrician exclaimed, standing near Vetkin. 'They opened the ash pit, let the steam out and gave our "guests" a hot welcome!'

The two Germans grabbed at their burnt faces and rushed off to the side. A German machine gun opened up and sprayed the cabin and tender. A second burst hit the lead carriage on an angle. There was no third burst, as the anti-aircraft guns of the train opened up a hail of lead onto the enemies on the platform, riddling the motorcycles and setting the fuel tanks alight.

Without slowing, the train passed the two blazing fires. The occupants of the headquarters carriage excitedly discussed what they had just witnessed.

'We have to see if anyone was injured when we were fired on,' Vetkin decided and gave a sign to Greenberg to follow him. The senior guide and Sosnovskaya hurried after the physicians.

It turned out that only the lead carriage was damaged. The German machine gun had knocked out half of the glass panes.

'You got us into the headquarters carriage just in time, Comrade Doctor,' the guide joked gloomily, looking at the holes in the doors of four compartments, 'otherwise half of the train team would have surely been killed.'

'Take out the broken glass and cover the windows with blankets,' Vetkin ordered.

'In two hours, we'll be in Slutsk. There we'll find some replacement planes,' the senior guide assured him. 'And maybe we'll get some other equipment. We have no big pots for cooking, and we need a stove and kitchen utensils.'

'They will give us all that,' Vetkin nodded in agreement. 'And now all of you go to your places. Aleksander Iosifovich and I will make our rounds.'

'A wounded soldier in the third carriage is complaining of a bad stomach ache,' Sosnovskaya reported with anxiety.

'Alright, we'll begin with him.'

The sergeant, wounded in the forearm, was pressing his hand to his stomach and breathing heavily.

'When did the pain begin to bother you?' the doctor asked compassionately.

'In the morning,' the sergeant answered, knitting his brow. 'Now it's very painful.'

Vetkin began to palpate the stomach and attentively watched the expression on the soldier's face. He thought for a moment, stripped the patient to the knees, and continued his palpating and observed the sergeant's groin area.

'At MacBurney's point12 there is severe inflammation, the muscles are tense on the right side. I believe you have observed Britten symptoms13,' Vetkin concluded, and looked at Greenberg for confirmation.

---

12   A painful point on the front of the abdominal wall.
13   A sign of acute appendicitis.

The surgeon nodded and said confidently, 'All told, I'd say we have an appendectomy here'

'It looks like that,' Vetkin agreed. 'Well, we'll check his temperature according to Vidmer14 just to be sure. Liza, take the sergeant's temperature in both armpits.'

The wounded soldier pressed the thermometer into the armpit of his healthy arm without a peep, but he looked at the doctors with doubt.

'Everything is all right, my friend,' Vetkin said and sat down next to the sergeant. 'A peacetime disease has struck you, appendicitis. We'll get rid of it.'

Addressing Greenberg, he said, 'Aleksander Iosifovich, get everything ready for the operation. Have Khomenko and a nurse help you.'

'I can go it alone,' the surgeon protested. 'I need the nurse, but Khomenko ought to stick to his planned duties. After all, the operation is routine.'

'Not really!' Vetkin objected and shook his head. 'It's not clear what the condition of his appendix is. I can assist you, if you don't mind.'

The senior guide said that it was an hour's journey to Slutsk.

'The two of us, I think, can manage it,' Vetkin commented on the news, and invited Greenberg to follow him. Then he spoke to the guide and the senior nurse, 'Prepare the patient and facilities for the operation.'

The doctors hurried to the headquarters carriage where there was an ordinary office desk, the only one in the train.

---

14   *A higher body temperature in the right armpit.*

As the procedure began, Vetkin watched the sure movements of Greenberg's hands, and felt the satisfaction of appreciating a fellow professional in action.

'He made an incision through MacBurney's point. Quite deftly, I should say,' he thought, holding an instrument out to the surgeon.

But Greenberg didn't take the instrument he offered, and instead used the end of the scalpel to move aside the hypodermic fatty tissue. Then, with his next movement, he smoothly cut the surface fasces, and then used Cooper scissors to cut the abdominal muscle tissue. He clamped the oblique and transversal muscle tissue.

A couple more sleights of hand and Greenberg pushed his index finger into the patient's abdominal cavity.

'He wants to see if there are any adhesions,' Vetkin thought.

Judging by the way the surgeon began to move the caecum15 to the wound, he understood that the incision location was over its dome. Soon after the dome of the caecum the appendix appeared through the wound.

The train slowed down. Master Sergeant Tarasenko entered the headquarters carriage and stood frozen at the door. Vetkin asked the senior nurse to assist the surgeon and turned to the sergeant.

'We are approaching Slutsk, Comrade Doctor,' Tarasenko sighed heavily. 'Everyone got a sandwich, but now we have neither bread, nor butter, and we have got little sugar. We need more food.'

Vetkin nodded and began to take off his coat, mask, and surgical gloves, thus transforming from a surgeon

---

15   *The first section of the large bowel.*

into the ambulance train commander. On their way to the lead carriage, he asked Tarasenko, 'How many sandwiches were given to the wounded, the medical staff, the conductors and the train crew?'

The first sergeant took a sheet of paper out of his tunic pocket and reported, 'Six hundred fifty-two sandwiches, two for each person.'

'How many did the wounded and the patients get?'

'Five hundred forty-six. Nobody went hungry, Comrade Doctor. In total there are two hundred seventy-three men and women.'

Vetkin was startled at the thought that in all the commotion, this was the first time he knew the exact number of wounded and patients on board.

The train began to slow down. Through the windows, single-storey log houses, half-covered with apple and cherry trees, sailed by. A dirt road appeared behind the houses. It was about thirty metres from the railway embankment. Along the road a continuous stream canvas-covered trucks moved slowly eastwards. They were making a lot of dust. Some of them were towing artillery pieces.

Some men on horseback trotted along the roadside, overtaking the trucks.

Women and children sat perched upon their carts loaded with their household possessions, as the men sat in front driving the horses along. But most of the refugees were fleeing the war on foot, with small bundles on their backs or with nothing, simply hoping for the best.

Vetkin, Tarasenko and the senior conductor stood in the passage of the lead carriage and watched the upheaval of war unfold.

The wind blew the black engine smoke into the windows, loosely covered with blankets. They had been smashed an hour ago by the German machine gun fire.

'Look, they are marching without any rifles! How are they going to fight?' Tarasenko exclaimed, breaking the silence and pointing to the road.

Puffing, the train overtook the long column of soldiers. The soldiers were marching, the tramp of their feet raising a cloud of dust. None of them had any weapons, only the three officers had pistol holsters on their belts.

'I hope they'll will be given weapons in Slutsk,' Vetkin said in a doubtful tone.

The ambulance train came up to the town station, passed the crowded platform and stopped near the water tower. About twenty men jumped down from the platform and rushed to the carriages.

Vetkin jumped out of the carriage and ran towards them, opening his gun holster as he moved.

'Stand back,' he yelled. 'This train is carrying wounded soldiers! Wounded only! Stand back! I'll shoot!'

Tarasenko ran up, pistol in hand. He shot twice into the air. Those who had jumped from the platform ran back, tripping over the rails.

Vetkin fastened his holster and headed back to the engine. Kuvaldin was slowly getting down from the cab. He tiredly waved his hand in answer to the silent question. He wiped his sooty forehead with his sleeve and said, 'I'll go see Vasilyev, the station master. We are old friends. I think he'll get us some trained boys for the locomotive crew. The trip, I see, is going to be a long one.'

'And how is Kalinich and his antiaircraft gunners?' Vetkin asked.

'Alright. One month of training and they'll be able to shovel coal as well as they can fire machine guns. Kalinich has run off to find food.'

'I have many questions for the local authorities, including the food problem. So let's go to the station master together, you can introduce me to him.'

Tarasenko and Sosnovskaya, notepad in hand, came up to them just then.

'You will stay here with the wounded,' Vetkin said, glancing at his subordinate. 'I appoint Greenberg as my deputy. If necessary, ask him. I'll soon return. Liza, examine the refugees carefully; see if any of them are sick. Examine everyone. Tell Khomenko to help you.'

It was noisy in Station Master Vasilyev's office. Without interrupting his telephone conversation, the broad-shouldered, dark-haired man raised his hand and greeted Kuvaldin with a short gesture.

'I understand!' he shouted into the telephone receiver, his rumbling baritone overpowering the any other sound. 'I do understand that it is urgent! I'll do my best!'

He hung up and embraced Kuvaldin.

'Hello, Slava! How did you get here?'

'With the ambulance train.' Kuvaldin nodded towards Vetkin. 'This is its commander. Feel free to introduce yourself.'

The station master rushed over to Vetkin. Shaking the doctor's hand with both of his, his loud voice once again filled the office.

'Divine Providence must have sent you here! Half an hour ago a column of trucks and staff cars left to the east. They've got many wounded men. Among them is the corps commander, Borin. He has a bad wound that requires urgent attention. You'll manage to catch up with them near Starye Dorogi.'

'We can still take more than two hundred wounded,' Vetkin said. 'But we need foodstuffs. If you help us get them from the warehouses...'

'The warehouses were destroyed by an air raid yesterday,' Vasilyev interrupted the doctor. 'They burnt down. The Germans have bombed the town repeatedly from the first day of the war. You must depart immediately. Do you hear the cannonade? Our troops are holding a line near Lyadno and Malyshevichy. I don't think they will last long, for this morning we received the order to evacuate.'

'Choose a team for the ambulance train, Slava. I'll not drive it any further,' Kuvaldin announced unexpectedly. 'My place is here. Will you take me as an assistant?'

'Did you drive the train yourself?' the station master asked his friend in disbelief.

'Yes, I did. It happened. We must put water in the tender. We need coal as well, and sand. God forbid we find ourselves skidding.'

'I won't leave without food!' Vetkin said sharply. 'The wounded and the refugees need food, as do the medical staff and train crew.'

Vasilyev threw up his hands in despair. Suddenly, his face brightened.

'I've got an idea. There is a grocer's two hundred metres from the railway. Requisition everything in the name of authorities. I'll give you a written order right away.'

The station master wrote something on a sheet of paper and thumped down the official stamp over his florid signature.

'Go ahead! I'll send the train crew to you immediately.'

Addressing Kuvaldin, he said loudly, 'Carry out your first order, Viacheslav, as my deputy. Ensure the ambulance train is sent off in the shortest possible time.'

On the platform, Vetkin and Kuvaldin shook hands, said a brief farewell and expressed their hope to meet again soon, 'As soon as we drive the fascists from our country.'

Kuvaldin headed for the depot, and Vetkin hurried to the hospital train. Near the carriage with the anti-aircraft guns Senior Lieutenant Kulinich was scolding a soldier. 'Are you a baby? You can't tell salt from sugar, can you?'

'Today's soldiers, Comrade Doctor,' he complained to Vetkin. 'The store saleswoman tells him to fill a bag with sugar, but he filled it with salt instead. It's a good job I chit-chatted with her. The woman softened up and gave me a packet of sugar as a present. She also gave me some bread, a big piece of butter, and some canned meat.'

'Is the shop far away?' Vetkin interrupted him.

'No, it's quite nearby, maybe one hundred and fifty metres away.'

'Take your soldiers and let's go.'

The food shop was really close to the railway. It occupied the ground floor of a building with a crumbling plaster façade. Two carts stood outside the entrance.

Vague noises and loud voices came from inside.

'Stay here, be ready for trouble,' Kalinich instructed the four soldiers and drew his pistol.

Vetkin followed him and took his weapon off safety. The officers stepped into the half-dark interior.

Four men in jackets and caps were collecting food, cigarette packets, bottles of wine and quickly stuffing it into sacks. Two salesgirls were crouching in the corner, crying silently with their faces in their hands.

The looters stood stock still when they caught sight of the officers, but only for an instant. Then they rushed for the exit. Shots rang out, and one of the thieves fell to the floor. A second man sank to his knees, holding his stomach, a few steps further.

'Fire!' Petrenko roared to the soldiers. A salvo from four rifles sent the two remaining runners to the ground.

'Who is the manager of this shop?' Vetkin asked the shop employees, who were wiping their tears with handkerchiefs.

Unable to speak, an elderly woman pointed to herself. Vetkin silently gave her the requisition order from the station commandant.

'Take them away so they don't interfere with the loading,' Kalinich ordered the soldiers and pointed at the bodies.

'One of them is groaning, Comrade Senior Lieutenant,' a tall soldier reported.

'Drag them out! Why are you standing still? Lay them all near the wall at the entrance. Get a move on. Faster!' Kalinich waved his hand.

'Thank you, officers!' the manager said as she came up to Vetkin. Those bandits just barged in and threatened us with knives.'

'There, there. It's all over. Help us pack up the food and open the storehouse. The paper says you must allow us to take everything to help the wounded.'

The soldiers loaded the carts with sacks, boxes, and packets. Kalinich, while filling a sack with tins, smiled and observed, 'Every cloud has a silver lining. A little dust-up netted us two carts. Otherwise we would have had to carry everything to the train on our backs.'

First Sergeant Tarasenko practically leaped for joy at the sight of the two carts piled high with supplies. Unable to contain himself, he blurted out, 'Would you look at that! We'll last another week on that for sure.'

'Ten minutes for unloading!' Vetkin ordered. 'The countdown has begun!'

A blond-haired youth ran up and introduced himself to the doctor, 'I am Kolentsev, assistant of the engine driver. The locomotive is ready to depart. When do we start?'

Vetkin glanced at his watch.

'At five forty-five. We must catch the motorized convoy with the wounded. It left town an hour ago. Can you catch up with it?'

The driver's assistant shrugged his shoulders and said, 'We'll try. We've got to meet them at the crossing in Starye Dorogi. That's the only place where the dirt road crosses the rails. We'll try to keep up maximum speed. The coal seems to be good. I think we'll get up to fifty kilometres per hour.'

Vetkin nodded and agreed, 'OK. Keep an eye out for a signal from the lead carriage. If we hang out a white cloth it means we have to stop.'

The young man hurried back to the engine.

The commandant dashed down the steps from the carriage tambour, which had been converted into a kitchen and pantry.

'It only took us ten minutes,' Kalinich reported, and wiped the sweat from his brow. He lit a cigarette and gave one to each of the soldiers who had helped with the loading. 'And where should we put our carts now, Comrade Doctor?' he asked.

'There are a lot of refugees on the platform. They won't all be able to catch a train. Offer the carts to them.'

The locomotive at the head of the hospital train whistled powerfully. The carriages began to move and, slowly gaining momentum, rolled away from the war.

To my mother, Antonina Stepanovna Kantonistova, veteran of the Great Patriotic War.

THE ARMY DOCTOR

'Toskas! It's war!' shouted wide-eyed Mishka Loginov, a student in the surgical department, as he rushed into the room at the Medical Institute dormitory.

Sitting at a table overloaded with books and notebooks, two fair-haired young women, both named Antonina ("Toska" for short), stared at him in surprise.

'What war? Are you kidding us again?' said Big Toska, the plumper of the two, with a dismissive wave of her hand. 'Don't bother us, we're preparing for the exams. Tomorrow we have an exam, and you know it.'

'F-o-o-l-s!' Mishka hissed intensely. 'It's war with the Germans! Molotov was on the radio. I was sent to inform everybody about it. All are to be present at the assembly hall at 2 p.m.'

Mishka wiped the sweat from his freckled forehead with the sleeve of his flannel shirt and ran out of the room to tell the others, his boots clumping down the corridor.

'W-a-r,' Little Toska pronounced in disbelief. 'And what about the exams, the institute and—?'

'The institute?' Big Toska grabbed the nearest textbook, "The Anatomy and Physiology of Eyesight." 'We'll keep on studying medicine. You see yourself as an ophthalmologist, don't you? And the Red Army will give

Hitler such a kick in the ass that he will limp back to Berlin.'

Little Antonina didn't share her girlfriend's optimism. 'It seems to me that everything will be different now,' she ventured.

'How do you know? It's in God's hands, as strange as that sounds for Komsomol members.16 You'd better tell me the parts of the juvenile tract in the eyeball.'

Near Theatre Bridge and Pushkin Square, gusts of wind swept the last withered leaves from nearly bare trees in the town park into the river Uvod. A lonely duck, separated from the flock that had already flown to warmer climes, circled over the dark wormwood. Thick, granular snow began to fall from the dense, low cloud cover, coating the thin ice on the river with a white blanket.

People hurried to the centre of the town along the bridge. Among them were those who intended to begin their studies at nine o'clock in the classrooms of about thirty town colleges and institutes.

The Ivanovo Medical Institute's foyer thronged with students. Teachers and students crowded near a big announcement, which took up nearly half the wall, and were attentively reading the slanting lines written in black Indian ink.

'In accordance with the October 20 declaration of a state of siege in Ivanovo and surrounding region, a working party will be formed. It will be sent to build defensive works. The team will consist of third – and fourth-year

16   Komsomol is the Russian abbreviation for the All-Union Leninist Young Communist League.

students and some teachers. There will be changes in the syllabus, and the students will be informed. The lists of team members will be available by 2:00 p.m. Everyone on the lists is to be in the assembly hall at 3:00 p. m. to receive instructions.'

The blasts raised clouds of sand and soil that, when they fell, painted the dazzling white snowy fields black. People with spades and picks jumped into the craters one by one or two by two. They threw the frozen chunks of soil out of the pit, westwards.

In one of the craters both Toskas were working. They had been digging the antitank ditch for five days and knew by now that first they had to throw out the big frozen chunks of sand, then shape the trench: four metres wide and two metres deep.

'Mishka said that the fascists have taken Volokolamsk,' Little Toska said as she took a breather and shook the dirt out of her felt boots.

'Had taken, not have taken!' Big Toska retorted as she angrily drove her spade into the bottom of the crater. 'Even if they take Moscow, their tanks will come up against our ditch and others like it!'

She took off her glove and rubbed her nose bitterly.

'It's not far from here to Kovrov. About one hundred kilometres as the crow flies, not more,' Little Toska sighed.

'We won't let the fascists into your hometown. Dig deep and they will get stuck here, you'll see.'

Having rubbed her nose warm, Big Toska picked up her spade and decisively thrust the polished edge into the slightly frozen ground on the side wall of the pit.

'Good girls!' said a foreman, his face red with cold, who looked down into the pit. 'Carts with wood will arrive by evening. We'll warm the earth and ourselves with bonfires.'

He sighed and said quietly, 'Even for men, this work is too hard, and not everyone can manage., For you, girls, it is a truly tough going. But there's no way round it–'

'It's not hard labour!' Little Toska interrupted the man. 'We're defending the Motherland!'

'But…it's just that you are very young…I'm sorry for you,' the man said, and waved his hand before hurrying to the next crater.

'Sympathetic type, isn't he?' Big Toska muttered and threw out some soil. 'We shall fight the fascists even more fiercely.'

'Soon enough,' her friend said, deftly straightening the western wall of the pit with her shovel. 'The sixth-year students left for the front three weeks ago.'

'Our turn won't be so soon. The fifth-year students write the state exams in January, ours are later. Well, my friend, let's have lunch.'

Nodding in agreement, Little Toska got out of the pit, took off her dirty mittens, rubbed her hands with snow, and took out a paper package from her quilted jacket pocket. She unwrapped it on her lap. Lunch consisted of two slices of brown bread and butter. The slices were frozen, but the hungry girls swallowed them in no time.

'Let's get to work!' Big Toska announced, jumped into the ditch and began to shovel earth onto the western lip of the crater.

'Borrow a pick from the neighbours,' she shouted to Little Toska, who was about to jump in.

By evening, the temperature had dropped. It took the young women about two hours to make the six kilometres to their billets in the last house near the river. The hamlet was named Shatry. Their tired bodies ached after the ten-hour workday.

Their host, a woman of sixty whom they called Gavrilovna, invited the two Antoninas to the table, poured some potato soup from a big cast-iron pot and pushed it over to the girls, saying, 'Help yourselves, please. It's fresh off the stove, still warm.'

Interrupting one another, the girls thanked the hostess and began to eat the plain hot soup with delight. After that, they lay down on the floor in the sleeping place prepared for them.

Their sleep was interrupted in the morning by Mishka, who had come to the house. He had been nicknamed "Info-Mishka" for bringing all the necessary and unnecessary news to the students in the village.

'It's time to finish our work, Toskas. The dean ordered me to inform everyone that tomorrow morning a new group is coming. We'll return to the institute in Ivanovo. Well, is this good news?'

Without waiting for an answer, he left the house.

The winter and spring of 1942 passed like a flash for the two Antoninas. That year, for the first time in the history of the institute, fourth-year students graduated. It took them four years instead of the usual six year to become physicians. Professors and teachers worked with the students from morning until night, including days off. The students worked hard not out of fear, but for love of their work. They all realized that the armies bleeding at the front needed their help.

The July sun was pouring light through the window panes on the fresh graduates, who had crowded into the long corridor of the building. The door opened from time to time, and the director, a tall grey-haired man, looked at a sheet of paper and loudly invited the next newly-minted doctor to enter his office.

'Antonina Kantonistova!' the man announced and glanced at the crowd.

'Here I am!' Little Toska shouted from the side and forced her way to the front row.

The institute directors and two army officers sat at the office table.

'Congratulations on your successful graduation!' the officer with two stripes on his collar tabs pronounced in a hard voice. 'The front badly needs your knowledge now. Are you ready to fight for the Motherland?' the major asked. He paused and looked searchingly into the eyes of the girl in front of him.

'Yes, Comrade Major,' Antonina answered quickly and laconically, according to military regulations.

'You are to go to location N. You'll be assigned to the North-Western front. Set out immediately. Here are your instructions,' the major said, and handed Antonina a small sheet of paper.

'Understood, Comrade Major,' Little Toska said quietly and began looking through the instructions.

'Invite the next one,' the major stated to the grey-haired pro-rector.

In the corridor, Big Toska was the first to reach Antonina. Her question came tumbling out anxiously: 'Where are they sending you?'

'To the North-Western front.'

'Aha. Well, I'll ask them to send me there too.'

But her requests didn't help. The officer was unyielding, admonishing, 'Do you listen to the Soviet Information Bureau? Do you know that the fascists are dying to get to the Volga? These days, friendship is not the basis for our decisions. We must save the Motherland, and that means that everyone must go where he or she is needed most.'

'You won't be alone there,' Antonina calmed Big Toska, though she herself was in tears. 'Mishka is also being sent to Stalingrad, and many others...we'll write one another.'

'I'll write you every day. Our four years together have gone by in no time at all,' Big Toska sobbed, and embraced her friend.

In the little tent, all things came in threes: three bunks, three home-made tables, three rough-hewn stools. Three officers turned to a slender blond girl, dressed in a new military uniform.

'Present yourself,' said the thin, black-haired officer with two rectangles on the tabs of his tunic.

'Comrade Doctor! Doctor Kantonistova at your disposal!' Antonina said loudly. She saluted smartly and took her folded order paper from her pocket.

'You've come just in time, Comrade Kantonistova,' the thin officer remarked. He stood up and came over to Antonina. 'My surname is Svechnikov. I am the head of the medical battalion. Tomorrow we expect…on the whole, there will be a lot to do from the early morning on.'

After a pause, he cracked his fingers and asked, 'What did you plan to be after getting your diploma?'

'An ophthalmologist,' Antonina confessed with embarrassment.

'That's fine. You'll treat people's eyes. But you will do so after our victory. These days, all the battalion doctors are surgeons. You'll join the operative-dressing platoon. Its commander is Galina Nikolayenko. She's been at war since the first day and she is an experienced doctor. You'll learn everything from her. Give your documents to the executive officer and talk to the commissar,' the battalion commander instructed, indicating to the officers seated at the table.

Suddenly remembering something, the commander looked at his watch, clenched his fist, swore in a low voice, and ran out of the tent.

Antonina handed her documents to the executive officer and turned to the table where an elderly officer with gray-haired temples was seated.

The officer moved his stool to the opposite side of the table and said, 'Would you like to sit?'

'Oh, no; no, thank you, I'll stand,' Antonina protested, but the officer insisted. 'I am not begging you. I am ordering you to get comfortable on the stool and listen to me attentively. Is that clear?'

'Yes, Comrade Battalion Commissar,' Antonina answered according to the rules, recognizing the tabs on the officer's collar.

'You know military ranks, that's good. I'll tell you something to help you understand our situation.'

The commissar smoothed the hair on his large forehead and, looking into Antonina's eyes, slowly began to explain that which, in his opinion, each new officer in the medical battalion ought to know.

'I think that you heard some information from the Soviet Information Bureau about the Demyansk pocket. The Germans are holding on to the pocket with all their might. From this area the enemy could launch a new offensive on

Moscow, if they manage to pull together enough reserves. The Red Army will try to liquidate this threat. Tomorrow morning our division, along with other troops, will begin an offensive.'

The battalion commissar drew a deep breath, paused, and said, 'This is the third try in the last month and a half. The Nazis are fighting desperately, trying to obey Hitler's order to hold on at all costs. Among the enemy troops in the pocket are the SS men of the "Death's Head" division.'

The commissar looked at Antonina and continued softly, 'Have I frightened you with this talk of a "Death's Head" division?'

'No, no, Comrade Battalion Commissar, I'd like all Nazi heads to be dead, and the sooner the better.'

'Ah, you've got a sense of humour! Let's shake hands to that!' the officer laughed and held out his hand across the table to Antonina.

The canvas flap at the entrance rustled, and in came the Medical Battalion Commander. He looked at Antonina and asked the commissar, 'Is everything alright with Kantonistova?'

Having received a positive answer, the commander addressed the executive officer, 'Call in the senior surgeon and the head of the evacuation department immediately.'

Turning to the commissar, he said, 'Things look rotten, Matvey Ivanovich. The corps commander hasn't given us a single additional ambulance. All the trucks, he says, have been taken for carrying ammunition. And we only have, as you know, two dilapidated ones at the disposal. Tomorrow we'll end up carrying the wounded to the hospital on our backs. If we have three or four hundred patients a day, we're done for. To hell with it!'

The battalion commander threw his cap onto the nearest bunk, sat down at the table and put his head in his hands.

'And you, do the following,' the commissar said quietly to Antonina, 'Go out and turn to the right. The first big tent is the therapeutic room. You can't miss it. Above the door there is a plywood sign.'

'They know about you there,' the battalion commander added, without looking up.

Antonina left the stuffy tent and breathed in the forest air. Dozens of fragrances mixed with the freshness of the July evening, none of which had anything to do with the war. The clouds, hardly seen in the sky, thickened. Gusts of wind brought the first drops of rain.

Antonina walked on and soon found the tent where

a white board with a green sign marked "Therapeutic" hung over the entrance.

In the centre of the tent, near a table covered with bed sheets, a woman in a military uniform was reprimanding three young men in white smocks. They were sitting with scissors in their hands.

'I don't know what you heard when I was instructing you. I repeat again: among the hundred patients, there are about thirty badly wounded. It means that their wounds are in their chests, stomachs, heads, or necks. In addition, there are arterial injuries. The rest have injured arms and legs. Such wounds, as a rule, are considered light and moderate. That's why red and blue plates are to be made according to that proportion. We don't use yellow and white plates any longer. Do you understand now?' she admonished them.

The three of them jumped from behind the table and answered loudly, 'Yes, Comrade Doctor!'

The woman waved her hand and turned her back to the tables. On seeing Antonina she didn't ask anything, but expressed her opinion as if to a person whom she had known for a long time, 'The young ones are greenhorns, the day before yesterday they arrived as replacements. Three of our experienced nurses were sent to the hospital the other day. The reason is clear: they suffered heavy losses there. The fascists, the swine, bombed the hospital. And tomorrow...did the battalion commander tell you anything about the present situation?'

'Yes, yes, he told me,' Antonina assured her. She liked the woman's confident manner as much as her big grey eyes and full, oval face.

'Galina, Galina Nikolayenko, platoon commander,' the woman said and shook Antonina's hand. 'Well, everything, you see now in this tent belongs to our operative-dressing platoon. The nurses are now in the sterilizing room. Soon they'll come here. We have five medical orderlies. Two of them are making trestles for stretchers. And you see three of them. They are peering at you instead of working,' the commander of the platoon finished her brief instructions.

'Let's go to the sterilizing room,' Nikolayenko said and headed for the exit, followed by Antonina.

'Wow, it's raining harder. Can you run? Follow me! Run!' Galina exclaimed. Without waiting for an answer, she ran to the right along a narrow path to the larger tent.

The large tent consisted of three tents connected together, each with separate entrances. The women, wet through, ran into the first one.

'We've got a new team member,' Nikolayenko announced to the young women in clean white smocks. The girls were working at the tables in the centre and around the perimeter of the tent. 'Doctor Kantonistova, or Toska,'17 The platoon commander looked at Antonina for approval and asked, 'Do you mind if I call you Toska?'

'Of course not. There is beauty in simplicity,' Antonia responded.

Nikolayenko laughed heartily and addressed a shapely brown-haired girl with almond-shaped eyes, 'Katyusha, my brilliant senior nurse, show us how the handwashing station has been prepared according to Spasokukotsky's rules.18 But first give us coats.'

17   More familiar form of the name Antonina.
18   Sergey Spasokukotsky (1870-1943), Soviet surgeon and member of the
Soviet Academy for Sciences.

'Everything is ready, Galina Petrovna,' the brown-haired woman replied and pointed to the bench with two wash basins.

'I see the basins, I'm not blind,' Nikolayenko said, and pulled the white coat over her shoulders. 'Show me the rest.'

The brown-haired girl shrugged her shoulders, took away the gauze cape from the nearest table and rattled off the list of items laid out: 'Soap, sterile brush, 0.5 % liquid ammonia, 5 % iodine solution, rivanol 1: 1000, 2 % potassium permanganate, 1 % chloramine, sterile napkins, ethyl alcohol, three-minute hourglasses.'

Turning quickly to the next table, she went on, 'Here are scissors for cutting hair, a razor, pain killers, boiled needles and a syringe for injections, and blood transfusion ampoules.'

Pointing at a container hung on a smoothly planed pole, she finished with a sigh, 'And water with antiseptic, twenty litres.'

'All right,' the platoon commander said briefly. 'I examined the operating theatre in the morning, but show it to Antonina, our new comrade-in-arms.'

The women went to a large tent, the walls and the ceiling of which were all covered with sheets. The senior nurse reached inside the darkness and turned on the light. Pointing at the ceiling, she said, 'The light is battery generated. Some tank crew gave them to us as a present. Now we have two. It's enough for five nights. Then our drivers take them for charging. And we also have reflector lamps.'

Mounted to the ceiling, automobile electric lamps lit the long tables in the centre of the tent quite brightly.

'Here we've got everything we need for two teams of surgeons,' Nikolayenko began to tell Antonina about the equipment of the operating theatre in an even confident voice. 'Each team has two tables. While an operation is being performed on one table, nearby the next wounded soldier is being prepared. It's a conveyor belt.'

The platoon commander's look became very serious.

'Otherwise it's impossible,' continued Nikolayenko after a moment's reflection. 'Once the fighting begins there is a stream of wounded soldiers. We have to perform operations day and night. So, all of us stand at the tables.'

Noticing Antonina's eyes had widened, she tried to reassure her, noting, 'You'll not be given a scalpel at once. First, you'll gain some experience in bandaging, then you'll assist with operations. I went through it as well. And now look around and remember where everything is.'

Pointing at the tables and boxes on the benches, Nikolayenko began to describe briefly how to use them. 'The tables are for solutions, blood transfusion, sterile instruments, for injections of blood serum…'

The canvas flaps at the entrance rustled, and a stout man with a coat over his shoulders walked into the tent. Glancing at Antonina, he reported to Nikolayenko, 'Comrade Doctor, the meeting in the commander's room will take place at twelve sharp. Comrade Captain Yezhov ordered me to inform all the authorities of the battalion,' the man's deep bass voice intoned.

'I hear, Skvortsov, I hear.'

Glancing briefly at his elegant wristwatch, the platoon commander asked, 'Is the additional set of stretchers ready?'

'Yes, it is, twenty-five units. I've been working on that all day.'

'All day… tomorrow will be easier for you. Well, you can go.'

When Skvortsov left, Nikolayenko said approvingly, 'The squad commander. He is a medical orderly from God. He looks like an awkward bear, but he outperforms everyone. But he likes this,' the commander said, and flicked herself on the neck.[19] 'We have to keep an eye on him.'

She looked at her watch again and said hurriedly, 'Well, Katya, show the doctor everything and explain in detail. Then you can find sleeping accommodation for her in the women's quarters and prepare something for supper. I'm off to the meeting. The "hedgehog" takes being late very seriously.'

Having waved farewell, Nikolayenko waved goodbye and disappeared out of the tent.

'Who is the "hedgehog"?' Antonina asked.

'The chief of the battalion headquarters. His surname is Yezhov, and our people call him "yozhik" (hedgehog). He is a quiet man, but when he lays into you, you won't soon forget him!'

Having thought a little, the nurse suggested, 'Let's go to the outpatients' clinic. I'll find you something to

---

19   *Amongst Russian speakers, a sign for excessive drinking.*

eat. I imagine you are hungry after travelling. Tomorrow morning you'll see our bandaging tent. It looks, by the way, much like this one.'

The summer rain, which had wetted the forest and the tents for half an hour, was coming to an end. Little drops of water, unseen in the night darkness, gathered into small pools that appeared here and there on the paths between the tents.

In the clinic tent, on both sides of the narrow passage, which began at the door and ended at the opposite wall, there were improvised walls, made from sheets that divided the tent into two halves, for men and for women.

In the women's section, Antonina sat down on a rough-made stool and stretched her legs with pleasure. Only now she felt the fatigue that came after the long, eventful day. The quick hands of Katerina prepared supper, and Antonina emptied a pot of warm porridge with stewed meat and sipped sweet tea that smelled of pine needles from a big aluminum mug.

Senior Nurse Katerina turned out to be so talkative, that a quarter of an hour later Antonina was fully up to speed with the ins and outs of battalion life.

'Our battalion chief is a real commander. He is fair, and that's very important. If someone is guilty, he'll punish him severely. But if there are a lot of wounded soldiers, he helps with everything: triage, bandaging, assisting the surgeon. He performs operations as well. Once he was operating on a badly wounded man when a German plane strafed our camp. Everyone was shouting, "To the forest! Carry out the wounded!" But the battalion commander didn't pay any attention. He told me to take the patient's pulse and prepare a needle with a thread. He continued operating until he finished. Later, we found six bullet-holes in the ceiling of the tent.'

'And you?' Antonina asked.

'I was assisting him.'

The clinic tent, which was used as a lodging place for the medical staff of the operative and bandaging platoon at night, gradually filled with people. Some nurses entered the women's section. Antonina had seen them in the sterilizing room. After eating, they began to lay the stretchers down on saw-horses to make space for a new bed.

'Will you spend the night here too?' a petite, black-haired young woman asked and took some bedding from the box in the corner of the tent.

'If you don't mind,' Antonina nodded in agreement.

'Why would we mind?' the black-haired girl said philosophically, and covered the stretchers with unfolded sheets. 'We are all on the same team.'

'What's your name?' Antonina asked.

'Rita. And you are Antonina, I guess. You are the new doctor, Galina Petrovna told us.'

'Where is she now? Is she still at the meeting?'

'No, the meeting was short,' Rita answered. She came up closer to Antonina and, bending to her ear, whispered with excitement, 'She is in the hospital ward. There is a soldier with a self-inflicted wound, so she—'

'What kind of wound?' Antonina asked in surprise.

'A man with a self-inflicted wound. He is one of

the ones who shoot themselves. They deliberately self-mutilate, to escape the front line.'

'Are there many of them here?'

'Not many. There are many of those who refuse treatment in the rear hospital.'

'And what do they do with such cowards?' Antonina asked, feeling tense. Rita made no reply. Katerina, who had settled under her blankets, answered instead, 'They are sent to divisional headquarters with a medical card after treatment. And on the card, the letter "s" is written in a particular spot. From headquarters, under escort, they are sent to the divisional prosecutor.'

'Do they execute them by firing squad?'

Katerina answered reluctantly, 'I don't know. We never see them again.'

The nurses and Antonina started getting ready for bed in silence.

Rita took off her tunic and bra. She began to gently wipe her shoulders with a gauze ball, and then did the same to her neck and small breasts with taught nipples.

'Eh, a stickler for cleanliness,' Dasha, a short plump nurse, teased her. 'You waste so much material! He will take you as you are. Give him a little hint.'

Abruptly snatching away the sheet curtain, Nikolayenko entered the tent. The expression on her face showed that the platoon commander was in a dour mood.

'Dasha,' she addressed the plump nurse. 'Pour me a bit of something.'

Galina mixed the vodka with some water and drank

it down, but turned down the offer of bread. Five pairs of eyes, ready to help, looked anxiously at the commander. Looking at Antonina, the commander asked her, 'Do you know about the boy who shot himself? He is in the hospital tent.'

She nodded.

'My girls couldn't hold their tongues. What can I say! Someday they'll suffer for it, God forbid.' Galina went on, 'The kid, Sizov, is only eighteen. His birthday was on the first of June. He was drafted into the Red Army. Then he had ten days of training and was sent to the front line. In his first battle, there was an artillery bombardment. He couldn't stand it. A shell landed in the trench. All the others were killed, but he was lucky. He was covered with soil and a little concussed. When he regained consciousness there was no one alive around him, and he was still being shelled. There were explosions, smoke, and fire everywhere. So he wounded himself in the shoulder.'

'His nerves failed him,' Antonina sighed. 'But all the same he ought to have gone on—'

'Ought to, ought to,' Nikolayenko roughly stopped her. 'Of course, he ought to have,' she continued more softly. 'His pillow is wet with tears. He gripped my hand and didn't let it go. "Send me back to the regiment in the morning. I'm not a coward and I'll redeem myself with my blood," He said. But as to sending him to the regiment in the morning? It's out of the question! His collar bone was splintered. He will stay here for at least a week.'

'And how did he do it, Galina Petrovna?' Rita asked, interested.

'I also asked him,' the commander said, and made a helpless gesture with her hands. 'It's difficult to reach a trigger if you rest the barrel against your shoulder. And nearby, not a single person was alive. He confessed that he had taken off his boot and pulled the trigger with his toe.'

'Inventive,' Dasha observed, and shook her head.

'Alright,' Rita hushed her. 'Life is unpredictable. It was kind of psychological crisis. Have you heard about it?'

'That's enough. Let's stop the discussion.' Nikolayenko said, got up and pushed her way to the wooden bunk. She took off her blouse and gave an order: 'Dasha, put out the lamp. Tomorrow our artillery – "the God of War" – will wake us up at the crack of dawn.'

The cannonade woke up the medical battalion just as the early July sunlight began to paint the fleecy clouds pink. They floated high in the cool sky at night, and the sun was about to appear over the horizon.

The artillery fire was so intense that the thundering blasts soon blended into a single menacing roar which filled up the landscape. It seemed it was that rumble, rather than the fresh morning wind, which shook the trees in the forest, struggled into the tightly drawn canvas of the tents, or caused the drying underwear to flap on the clothes lines in the clearing.

Doctors and nurses, medical orderlies and assistants, cooks and drivers – the whole staff of the battalion left the tents and began their morning toilet. Captain Yezhov's loud voice kept them moving quickly. He stood near the commander's tent in his polished boots and neatly pressed and tucked uniform.

'Roll call in twenty minutes, be ready to fall in.!' he shouted.

Near the long washstands, the men washed in their underpants. When they'd finished, they rubbed themselves vigorously with stiff towels. The women, naked but for their bras and underpants, carefully soaped their arms and shoulders, and rubbed their bellies and necks with wet towels.

'Take off your tunic,' Nikolayenko said as she drew Antonina to the washstand. 'Once the action starts, you'll only have time to wipe your face and hands with some gauze, that's it. There's a free spot, let's go!'

Following the commander's advice and trying not to look at anyone, Antonina quickly took off her tunic and took her place near the washstand.

'Bat-t-a-l-ion!' glancing at his watch, the executive officer gave the order to fall in in a booming voice. The battalion staff lined up on a narrow path in front of the battalion tents.

'Line up by platoon. The right wing is for the reception and sorting-out platoon. Five steps between you. Fall in!'

The executive officer waited until the last soldiers had washed, dressed, and occupied their places in their platoons. Then he shouted, 'Right dress! Attention! Eyes left!'

Suddenly it became so quiet that the soldiers heard the sound of water falling into a tin washbasin.

The battalion commander and the middle-aged commissar came up to the battalion. Antonina knew them.

The commissar wiped his forehead with a gauze kerchief.

'At ease, at ease,' the battalion commander waved his hand to Yezhov, who was going to present himself. Looking at his colleagues, Svechnikov briefly gave them their mission. 'The artillery, as you can hear, has finished its work. In an hour, maximum in an hour and a half, the wounded will be brought here. We'll act according to Suvorov's principles: every one of us must know his role.[20] I have no doubts about those who have done this before. Those who have not will have to follow the instructions of the experienced doctors and nurses without any objections. And now listen to the commissar,' he pronounced.

The battalion commissar looked over the ranks and confidently said, 'The preparatory bombardment is over, and now the soldiers of our division are going to attack the Germans. I'm sure that this time the enemy will be crushed. We won't let down those who are now storming the German fortifications. We'll be fighting for the lives of Soviet Army soldiers, and there'll be no time to feel sorry for ourselves. We must be well-organized, efficient, and if necessary, support each other. As the inhabitants of Latium said, "Where there is consensus, there is victory".' The commissar finished his brief speech and glanced at the battalion commander.

'Dismissed!' Svechnikov intoned, and quickly headed for his tent, with a gesture motioning along the chief of staff Yezhov.

'Is the commissar also a medical professional?' Antonina asked while following Nikolayenko.

---

20   *Aleksander Suvorov (1730-1800), Russian military hero of the 18th century.*

'Yes, and a good one! He was the head of the surgical department in a Moscow hospital. His two sons were officers who served in the same division. Both were killed a year ago near Vyazma. That's when Matvey Ivanovich volunteered to serve at the front. He is fifty-four now.'

'What's his surname?'

'A famous name in medicine: Pirogov.'

In the tent labelled "Dressing Room," the whole operative-bandaging platoon had gathered.

'I don't see Skvortsov,' Nikolayenko asked the senior nurse. 'Where is our Hercules?'

'On the edge of the forest. Yesterday he cut wood like a like a real lumberjack. Not a single log fit into the stove. Now he is cutting the logs into smaller pieces.'

'Understood, Dasha, and now run to the triage room. Find out whether the ambulances were sent to the regiment's medical centre or are still waiting. And why are our new first-aid nurses lolling about? All three can run to the forest and fetch everything Skvortsov has cut, quickly. Move it! Take some ground-sheets. How else will you carry the firewood?'

Rita rushed into the tent with a frightened look on her face; her white nurse's kerchief was pushed to one side. She stumbled and fell on the arms of Antonina and Katya, who tried to steady her.

'What's the matter? Is there a fire under your behind?' Nikolayenko pounced on her. 'You'll break everything in here.'

'Galina Petrovna,' Rita panted. 'Sizov has disappeared from the therapeutic room.'

'What do you mean "disappeared"?' the platoon commander exclaimed, balling her fists. 'Did you look for him?'

'In all the tents. And he is not in the forest near the kitchen.'

'And in the men's latrines?'

'He isn't there either. All of them were open, except one. I shouted his name, but another voice answered...'

'He might have gone to his regiment,' Antonina said with an expressive look at Nikolayenko.

'Maybe, such things happen. Or maybe he has deserted and has gone to the rear.'

The platoon commander sighed and said, 'We'll have to report this to the authorities. What a fool! Three days ago we took him out of shock. What will he do with one arm at the front line?'

Keeping silent for a minute, she marched towards the exit and said, 'Kantonistova can fill in for me. Prepare boiling water and sterilize the surgical instruments.'

'What a mess!' Rita moaned, and shook her head in distress. 'Now Galina Petrovna will get a tongue lashing. Oh, she'll be dressed down by the battalion commander.'

'Don't complain!' Katerina interrupted her, 'Svechnikov is a just man, he'll understand...perhaps our man with the self-inflicted wound is somewhere nearby, maybe he'll be here soon.'

The young medical orderlies entered the tent with armfuls of wood.

'One thing off the list! Put them into the corner.'

The senior nurse put the surgical instruments on the

table with a pleased look, turned to Rita and said, 'Prepare some boiling water, and don't spare the wood.'

Barely heard somewhere in the distance, the rumbling noise of engines drove almost all the personnel of the medical battalion out of the tents. Two hundred eyes watched the forest road, which began near the tents and disappeared behind a sharp turn. The noise of automobile motors came from there.

'What is this? A circus performance?' Svechnikov bellowed. Antonina did not know that he had a such a thundering voice.

The medical battalion staff quickly returned to their positions in their tents.

'Triage team, get ready!' the battalion commander boomed. 'The rest, forward march and occupy your places! Get ready to for the arrival of the wounded!'

The trucks appeared from around the bend and approached slowly, slip-sliding in the uneven ruts.

'Two of them are our trucks; one belongs to the regimental medical point and one more, two...five trucks!' said the executive officer, Yezhov. He looked at his watch and noted the time of arrival on a pad. 'They are carrying about seventy men, maybe more.'

'We have our work cut out for us,' Svechnikov said sharply.

He had understood the instant he saw the trucks that his subordinates would have to endure a greater influx of wounded than they'd ever experienced before. Now he wished only one thing – that his battalion could meet the challenge like a well-oiled machine, run by an experienced master.

The five trucks crawled into the clearing and backed up to the tents.

A stocky lieutenant jumped out of the first ambulance and ran up to Svechnikov. He saluted and made to speak, but the battalion commander spoke first, asking, 'How many? What kind?'

'Sixty-three. Eleven badly wounded. There are some with tourniquets.'

'How are things up there? Are we advancing?'

The lieutenant shook his head negatively. Speaking in low tones, he unwillingly confessed, 'The Germans are standing firm. Counterattacking.'

Everyone lent a hand to unload the trucks: nurses, drivers, and medical assistants. The commander himself, along with the executive officer, began to help the nurses, like orderlies, as they both realized that the most important role was now to be filled by the senior surgeon, Aron Girson. Girson, though their subordinate, was responsible for examining and triaging the wounded. Tall and brown-haired, wearing round glasses, he looked over every arrival and decided on his lot with staccato orders:

'Shock. To Nikolayenko.'

'To the operating theatre. Cito.'[21]

'Bandaging.'

'To be evacuated to the rear.'

The stretcher-bearers put down the stretchers on the grass in rows and tried

to place the wounded in the shade to shelter them from the hot July sun.

---

21   *"Quickly" in Latin.*

The nurse, following the surgeon, quickly wrote down the instructions, stuck multicoloured tokens on the men's tunics and showed the stretcher-bearers where to carry them.

Soon they finished unloading the trucks. The commander of the receiving – and-sorting platoon, Letunov, a lean fair-haired man, signed the documents presented to him by the lieutenant in charge of the ambulance column. Letunov then said anxiously, 'Nine soldiers must be evacuated to the field hospital: those with wounded eyes, craniums, and one with a crushed jaw. All of them are in bad condition.'

Pointing at two trucks which were turning around, he asked the lieutenant, 'Do you know where they are bound?'

'No, I don't. The shells were unloaded at the warehouse, and as usual every empty vehicle must transport the wounded. I think they will go to the army depots.'

Without listening to the lieutenant, Letunov jumped onto the footboard of the departing truck. A round-faced officer with black stripes on his lapels was sitting near the driver. The truck put came to a sudden stop.

'Listen to me, acrobat,' the round-faced man said in a friendly tone. 'Next time I won't stop, and you'll have to travel on the footboard all the way to the positions at Kozin.'

'Oh, that's near the field hospital!' Letunov said happily. 'Take the badly wounded there, nine men, I beg of you.'

The broad-faced officer seemed to be pondering something.

'We've already helped you, and we've got definite instructions not to deviate from the route. We are an exception. Have you heard the song "Apple trees and pear trees were beginning to blossom"?'

'He means the new secret rocket launcher units, "Katyushas,"' Letunov understood, catching the officer's drift. 'They must be heading to the warehouse to transport shells for them.'

'Can you give our regards to "Katyusha"?' The platoon commander asked, making a gesture familiar to every military man.

'Of course,' the broad-faced soldier said in a lively tone. 'Open the back, Mikheev!'

The rocket supply unit officer took some medicine from Letunov and assured him, 'I'll get everyone to the destination, you needn't worry.'

Svechnikov came up. Looking at the departing trucks, he said, 'So, the captain agreed to take the evacuated soldiers after all. Well done!'

'That's right, Comrade Major, he agreed,' Letunov answered briefly and spat into the dirt.

'How many serious cases are left?' asked the battalion commander.

'Four pneumothorax, five fractures, an abdominal cavity, larynx, bladder…plus eleven soldiers are in a state of shock. Thirty-three,' Letunov said.

'Just like in Pushkin's fairytale,' Svechnikov said with a smile. 'We'll make bogatyrs of them yet.[22] If you need

---

22   *Bogatyrs is a hero of old Russian legends known for their strength.*

me, I'll be assisting Girson. Check on the distribution of rations. There are dark clouds in the sky. A reserve tent is to be pitched in case it rains. Send the lightly wounded out, they shouldn't wander from tent to tent and disturb those who are working.'

Having given these instructions to Letunov, the battalion commander walked to the operating theatre.

The wounded suffering from shock were placed in a separate ward on mattresses and covered with sheets.

'Let's get at the shock cases,' Nikolayenko gave orders from the last table of the bandaging room. 'Stretcher-bearers, start bringing them in. Skvortsov will be responsible. Carry the first man to me. The second table is Antonina, the third is Katya, Dasha will assist. Don't undress the wounded until they have been examined. Patients in shock are to be covered with two blankets.'

'Where did you get your operating experience?' Galina asked while watching Antonina transfuse blood.

'In Ivanovo. It was in November last year, when the wounded were brought there from the front. Before dinner we attended lectures, and then all of us went to the hospitals. At that time, we began to assist with simple operations.'

'Oh, Galina Petrovna! My patient isn't breathing!' Katya said as she feverishly tried to find the young soldier's pulse.

'Dasha, transfuse the blood to my patient!' Nikolayenko quickly turned to the wounded man who was nearly gone. She raised his eyelid, looked into the pupil and shouted, 'Skvortsov! Come here! Quickly!'

The man appeared in the tent with unexpected swiftness. He understood the brief gesture of the commander and put his big hand on the chest of the wounded soldier.

Nikolayenko picked up a piece of gauze, covered the soldier's face, but quickly removed it. She opened the soldier's mouth and muttered under her breath, 'The tongue is alright, thank God!' She inhaled deeply and sent the first breath of air into the lungs of the lifeless patient.

The rhythmic efforts of the platoon commander together with the powerful compressions of the corpsman did their work successfully. A minute later the pale face of the wounded soldier began to turn pink.

'It's time to stop nursing you, young man,' Nikolayenko said after taking his pulse. She stood up and added, 'Other soldiers are waiting for their turn. Katya, you can take it from here. Skvortsov, send the next one,' she ordered the medical orderly, when she saw Antonina finishing the transfusion.

'This one has wounds in both legs. Can we examine him?' Antonina glanced at Galina.

'We can, of course, but others in shock are waiting, and there are about thirty soldiers outside. Take off his trousers.'

The two bandages above the man's knees turned out to be saturated with blood, and the additional one on the right leg was soaked through as well. When Antonina took it off, she gasped. Nikolayenko turn to her.

'They've left the instrument in, they've forgotten to take it out!' Antonina pointed at the curved styptic forceps in the wound.

'They haven't forgotten,' the platoon commander glanced at the open wound and calmed her down. 'The injured vessel is too big, that's why it was blocked with the forceps at the regimental medical point. Though these forceps injure the tissue even more, they also stop bleeding more effectively.'

'What are we to do with him?' Antonina asked Nikolayenko.

'What to do, what to do! Same as the others: stop him from dying,' she said sharply. 'But he will take us an hour and a half, at least. That's enough time to treat all the patients in shock.'

The battalion commissar entered the bandaging tent. While tying up the tapes of his smock, the commissar pronounced, without referring to anyone in particular, 'Do you accept bald-headed men?'

'Matvey Ivanovich, my dear!' Nikolayenko threw her hands up happily. 'Just in time! We are in a jam, a lot of injuries!'

'Well, well, calm down, Galina Ivanovna, there'll be time for pleasantries later.'

The commissar looked over the tables, sized up the situation and approached Antonina.

'Go to the patients suffering from shock. I'll manage here alone.'

Turning to Dasha, he ordered, 'Give the disinfectant and tampons to me.'

While taking a tampon soaked in disinfectant, he remarked, 'I prepared my hands in the sterilizing room, but when I was walking through the tent, my smock became untied. So it won't do any harm to wash my hands again.'

Pirogov caught himself thinking that his explanations were superfluous, as the nurse was not a newcomer in the battalion and understood well why her hands should be well prepared for the operation.

The commissar, with his hands held up at head level, approached the table on which the soldier with the leg wounds lay. However, Commissar Pirogov was no longer there in that room. In his place stood a surgeon dressed in a white coat, ready to fight for the life of the wounded soldier.

'The shrapnel wound was cleaned properly,' he remarked, correctly diagnosing the type of wound. He then addressed the nurse, saying, 'See what injections he was given at the regimental medical point.'

Dasha was already holding the man's card and answered quickly, 'They gave him several injections, Matvey Ivanovich: antitetanic, and antigangrene serum, and morphine.'

'Clean the operating field with alcohol, and let's start according to regulations,' Pirogov said, before adding, 'lege artis.'[23]

The wounded man suddenly opened his eyes and groaned loudly.

'This is not the time to come to, my friend,' Pirogov remarked in a displeased tone. He felt the soldier's pulse and asked the nurse, 'What anesthetic have we got?'

'Chloroform, chlorethyl, ether...'

'No chloroform. The soldier has low blood pressure,

---

23   Latin, meaning "state of the art" or according to the latest scientific knowledge.

prepare some ether.'

Pirogov held his arms in the ready position and gave Dasha a look that meant for her to hurry.

Just then Letunov poked his head into the tent and blurted out, 'Comrade Commissar, the Army hospital phoned. They have already sent two trucks to take our lightly wounded. Our ambulance cars are finishing loading wounded men from the regimental medical points. They are due in half an hour.' Catching his breath, he added anxiously, 'It's going to rain soon.'

'Settle everything with the executive officer,' Pirogov ordered after listening to the commander of the receiving-sorting platoon. 'Don't bother the battalion commander without any reason. He and Girson are operating on badly-wounded soldiers, and we are also busy. We must manage to do our work: in half an hour the next group of wounded will arrive. Take all the bed cases to the hospital and therapeutic wards. All the rest should be sent to the reserve tent. Don't distract me any further.'

Letunov's head disappeared. Raindrops began drumming on the roof of the tent.

'The last one, Galina Petrovna,' boomed the thick bass of the commander of the sanitary department, filling the bandaging room. Skvortsov and his colleague carefully placed the wounded man onto the table.

Nikolayenko nodded.

'See if all the soldiers in shock have been given hot food, and give them sweet tea. The nurses must stay with them all the time.'

Looking at Antonina, she ordered, 'Take care of the

wounded. Examine everyone, change the bandages if necessary. Use morphine while bandaging only in a worst-case scenario. We are short of it. You'd better stir fifty grams of spirits into the water and give them a drink.'

'But Galina Nikolayevna, we have very little spirits left,' Katya said while wiping the table with a gauze napkin. 'Letunov took two pots of it'

'How did that happen? When? What right did he have to do that?' the platoon commander said indignantly.

'An hour ago. He said he needed it for work.'

'What work? I'll tell the commissar!' Nikolayenko shouted angrily, forgetting that the battalion commissar was operating two steps away from her.

Galina's shouts prevented Pirogov from doing his work. Holding a Reverdin's needle,[24] he turned around, came up close to Nikolayenko and said something through his mask.

The platoon commander said to Antonina, 'As soon as the alcohol comes to an end, use aviation gasoline to wash wounds.'

An orderly entered the tent, followed by a soldier with a red moustache. He had three triangles on his collar. His right arm was in a sling. The soldier informed everyone in a loud voice, 'They let me come in out of turn. I am the foreman of the company. They bandaged me in the battalion, but I fell down and passed out. I came to when I was in the ambulance. I have to be back as soon as possible. Gusakov is a temporary–'

'Comrade Foreman,' Nikolayenko interrupted him, frowning. 'We'll make a decision after we examine you.

---

24   *Surgical needle for suturing with an eye, which can be opened or closed by means of a slide.*

Don't speak so loudly, there are patients being operated on here.'

'Sorry, sorry,' the sergeant continued in whisper, 'but I desperately need to return to the company. I am supposed to give food and drink to everyone, and deliver ammunition, but Gusakov is very slow…'

'Not everything is so simple with the foreman,' Antonina thought, while she was unwinding his bandages, saturated with blood.

Her suspicions proved well founded. There were two bullet wounds in his arm.

When Dasha came up to her, Antonina said, 'Into the triceps and brachioradial, it's good that it is right through. It looks like the tendon hasn't been injured. Fetch some tampons with antiseptic and the blood transfusion gear.'

'You've lost a lot of blood,' Antonina said mildly to the senior sergeant.

'That's why you lost consciousness. You'll have to stay here a few days.'

Nikolayenko, Katya, and Rita joined the others in bandaging the wounded. Dasha, assisting Pirogov, beckoned to Antonina with her finger.

'Antonina,' the nurse whispered pleadingly, 'I must run to the forest, I can't stand it, will you replace me?' Antonina nodded and took her place. Outside there was the noise of engines again.

'The hospital trucks must have arrived,' Nikolayenko surmised, and then shouted, 'How many wounded left to be examined, Skvortsov?'

'Four, Comrade Doctor,' his voice rumbled in return.

This time the executive officer was responsible for the casualty transfer.

'Lightly wounded men, move quickly to the trucks! Keep order while you get in! Doctor Krylenko will accompany you.'

After counting the wounded that were ready to leave, Yezhov said to the nurse from the hospital, 'Check the papers of those who are leaving again.' Then he stopped a medical orderly who was running by and asked, 'Where are the thermoses for the evacuated soldiers? Run and fetch them.'

After that he reminded Krylenko, the tall, thin therapist of the hospital company, 'Don't forget to return all the blankets. And come back as soon as possible by any passing truck. Very soon the next group will be brought in from the front line. Here they are now,' the executive officer threw up his hands. 'Speak of the devil.'

The battalion ambulances had appeared on the forest road.

'No time to have a smoke,' Yezhov said in distress, and addressed the doctors and nurses who had walked out of the hot tents for a breath of fresh air, 'To your places, comrades!'

'How many have we got this time?' he asked Letunov, who had met the column.

'According to the documents, thirty-four. We'll see if they're all still alive,' the senior lieutenant answered laconically.

The senior surgeon left the operating theatre, straightened his shoulders, stretched his neck, and once again assumed the primary role in the battalion. He began to triage the wounded, a familiar process by which he, surgeon Girson, determined the fortune of every wounded soldier: to live or to die.

The executive officer decided to distract the senior surgeon from his work for a moment, 'Aron Moiseevich, how is the battalion commander getting on?'

'Perfectly fine, he is operating,' the surgeon answered briefly and quickly headed towards the wounded, who were lying on stretchers.

The sun burned brightly and heated the air in the battalion tents to very high temperatures. The four small gauze-covered windows of the bandaging tent did not help much.

'To the "dressing room"! Katya begins,' Nikolayenko ordered. The senior nurse hid in the entrance of the tent. Seeing Antonina's surprise, the platoon commander explained, 'Our underclothes are soaking wet. Take everything off, and work in your white coat. Otherwise you'll faint, it's happened before.'

There were only four cases of shock this time. But there were more serious wounds. After receiving the information from the nurse, who wrote down the results of the leading surgeon's triage, Letunov ran to the executive officer. Yezhov was sternly admonishing the medical orderlies, who were standing at attention, 'You must be able to do many things. All the nurses are busy now with bandaging and assisting operations. Take the cups and give all the bed-ridden soldiers some water to drink, excluding those with abdominal issues. On the double!'

The executive officer turned to Letunov and said, 'Situation report! Are there many badly wounded?'

'Twenty-six. Four of them are in shock. Three require amputations. Two craniocerebral cases. Five have collapsed lungs.'

'Understood,' Yezhov said and stopped listening. 'We'll bring in the whole hospital company. I'll give the orders, and you get busy with those who will be evacuated.'

'My goodness! Again?' Letunov exclaimed and pointed at a dusty cloud approaching the place along the forest road.

'Just two passing trucks,' he said, after looking carefully at the approaching vehicles.

The wounded from the front line were delivered more and more frequently. Their arrival became a continuous flow of wounded human bodies to the place where people who had given the Hippocratic oath tried with all their strength to help.

All the doctors and nurses of the hospital company joined in operating and bandaging.

'Hello!' Ivan Fadeev said as he appeared in the bandaging tent. He was a blue-eyed blond doctor from the hospital company. Winking at Nikolayenko, he joked, 'I've been sent by the executive officer to support you. Therefore, I'm entirely at your disposal.'

'Report to the commissar, Ivan,' Galina responded listlessly, without responding to the joke. 'He is operating at the first table.'

Pirogov momentarily interrupted operating on a wounded soldier, nodded to the therapist, and said something into his ear.

'The commissar said that you would give me a place to operate,' Fadeev told Galina.

'Alright, just wait a minute.'

The medical orderlies moved some tables around and set up an operating station.

The doctor strode up to the commissar with a pot in his hand. Raising his gloved hands, covered with blood, Pirogov walked to the corner of the tent. Fadeev followed him.

'What is going on?' Antonina thought, surprised at his actions, which she'd caught out of the corner of her eye. She bent over the wounded soldier.

Two stretcher-bearers laid a bandaged soldier on the table.

'Take the pot,' Fadeev told one of the stretcher-bearers.

Antonina glanced at her colleague and gasped in surprise – she had seen the glass filed with yellow liquid. 'Urine,' she guessed silently. 'Pirogov didn't want to waste time sterilizing his hands again.'

Antonina looked at the others. They kept on working without paying attention to the – for them unremarkable – episode. Fadeev took of his coat and headed for the sterilizing tent.

Nikolayenko began to give orders:

'Rita, you'll work with Fadeev, prepare the patient for his operation.'

'Tonya, finish bandaging and come here, you'll assist me.'

'A drink! Give me some water!' a wounded soldier on a stretcher shouted loudly.

'Give him a wet napkin!' the platoon commander ordered.

Rita quickly wetted a piece of gauze in water, folded it and put it in the man's mouth.

'Clench it in your teeth and suck. Don't drink, you'll die if you do. Try to endure the thirst,' the nurse informed him.

Moving backwards so as not to touch the canvas entrance flaps with his disinfected hands, Fadeev appeared in white medical clothes. He winked encouragingly at the nurse. Rita answered with a quick nod and smiled. She liked the broad-shouldered, good-natured man and didn't keep it a secret. The doctor came up to the stretchers and examined the wounded soldier.

'Many shrapnel wounds. Rita, prepare the blood transfusion equipment. He is in a pre-shock state. He's lost at least a litre of blood. What is his blood type? Check his card for the time of wounding.'

'It's been nearly six hours, Comrade Doctor,' the nurse answered quickly. 'I've just looked at it.'

'Then hook up the transfusion kit, I'll do the preparations myself.'

By the evening, Antonina couldn't feel her legs. They were so leaden that she had to clench her teeth to carry on with the work. At one point she probably lost consciousness for a moment, because she heard the sharp and displeased voice of Nikolayenko shouting, 'Richter! Richter scissors, I say!'[25]

Antonina gave the scissors to Galina and realized that her strength was about to give out. Nonetheless, through sheer willpower she forced herself to remain upright.

25   A type of surgical scissors.

'Commissar Matvey Ivanovich is twice my age, but he hasn't left the operating table,' she reproached herself, looking at Pirogov preparing for a leg amputation. He was holding an arc saw and looking at it intently. Out of nowhere, Nikolayenko's hand appeared holding a tampon.

'Antonina, your nose is bleeding!' Galina said. 'Take a two-hour rest. That's an order. Get dressed, the nights are cool here.'

Plodding along with difficulty, Antonina left the tent. The setting sun touched the tops of the pine trees, and the stuffiness of the tent was replaced by the freshness of a light wind. Around the tent, the wounded were lying side by side and waiting for their turn to be operated on. The nurse was walking the stretchers with a mess tin.

Antonina nearly fell as she entered the forest, but steadied herself against a birch trunk.

'Just think, an army doctor', she told herself, 'I'm so weak on account of the stuffy air in there. You must endure, Antonina, at any cost.' She smiled ruefully and thought, 'The mind is willing, but the body is weak.'

'Comrade Doctor, let's walk to the ambulatory,' the senior nurse suggested. She had appeared suddenly, goodness knows where from.

'There is tea and buckwheat porridge.'

'Katya, you can call me by name,' said Antonina weakly, and released the tree.

A growing noise, loud and peculiar, made the women stop. Streaks of flame tore across the scarlet sky.

'Katyushas!' the nurse said and clapped her hands. 'Give our regards to the fascists! Particularly from me, I might add.'

In the ambulatory, after swallowing two spoons of buckwheat porridge with margarine, Antonina collapsed onto the packages of bandaging material and fell asleep at once. It seemed that she had only slept a moment when Nikolayenko roused her.

'Come to my table. Katya is there already.'

Rita called her over as she entered the bandaging tent. Fadeev, from the hospital company, stood at his operating station and was trying to make out what the wounded soldier lying on the stretcher was saying.

'Do you speak German?' the nurse asked. 'This is a German captive. He has an abdominal wound.' Antonina nodded.

Fadeev stepped aside and turned his back to Rita. He took off his mask and said to Antonina, 'The executive officer accompanied this German in person, so your hide is on the line here. The captive is supposed to be from Ravushevo. He could have valuable information. He is trying to tell me something, but all I can get is "bitte, bitte."[26] It's harmful for him to speak, by the way.'

Shaking his head, he added angrily, 'Many of our boys are waiting their turn. And we'll need two hours for this German.'

Antonina had had an easy time with the German language at school and at the institute. She easily remembered new words, pronunciation rules, word order, and verb tenses.

The German tried to speak again but wheezed so heavily she missed it.

'Noch einmal bitte,'[27] Antonina asked the captive to

---

26   German for "please, please."
27   "Once again, please" in German.

repeat, which he managed to do. Then she interpreted: 'He begs that a Russian doctor save his life. He says that German doctors don't bother operating on stomach wounds. He has three children, and he did not want to fight.'

'Tell this pacifist to shut up, otherwise we'll leave the shrapnel where it is,' Fadeev said sharply.

Antonina came back to the table where Katya was preparing a junior lieutenant, wounded in the shin, for an operation.

'Nikolayenko has just gone to get some rest,' Antonina tried to explain the situation to her. 'Who will–'

'We will,' the nurse said flatly. 'Don't worry. I studied at the medical institute in Minsk for two years. And here I got some surgical experience. It took me half a year. I assisted some doctors. Not long ago I was allowed to operate on my own, except for complicated cases.'

Katya drew some liquid into a syringe, sprinkled a little aside, and deftly made a hypodermic injection.

'Novocain,' she said to Antonina, 'the fragment isn't deep, we can operate on this one using local anesthesia.'

Behind the tent they heard the roar of an approaching truck.

'Well, replacements have arrived by ambulance,' Katerina surmised correctly. 'Usually there are about fifteen.'

Suddenly they heard shouts, swearing and threats outside. The commissar ordered the assistant to finish 'sewing up,' took off his mask and bloody gloves and hopped outside.

Near the ambulance that had just arrived, a tall, thin captain with a bandaged neck and the Red Star order on his tunic was shouting and gesticulating in Letunov's face: 'You want us to turn around? My goodness! I'll turn you around, mark my words!'

'Stop quarrelling!' an officer in a bloodstained coat yelled and ran up to the two. Pirogov addressed them in a steely tone that brooked no objections: 'A major is talking to you! What is the problem!'

Looking at the commissar's coat, the wounded officer lowered his tone and said gloomily, 'Twenty-two wounded, three badly. They're from N brigade, and managed to escape encirclement by trudging through the marshes, without food.

'Do you see those stretchers?' the commissar interrupted the captain and pointed at the wounded soldiers lying near the tents. 'There are nearly fifty soldiers waiting to be operated on.'

Then he said in a lower tone, 'Even then, not all of them will live to see the operating table.'

The captain sighed with understanding, silently saluted, and opened the door of the cab.

'Wait,' Pirogov called him. 'We'll take the badly-wounded. You can take the rest to your division's medical battalion. Senior Lieutenant Letunov will show you the road until the second fork. From there, just follow the signs.'

The medical orderlies unloaded the serious cases. Letunov stood on the step of the truck, and the ambulance started off. Its headlights pierced the darkness, a moving swathe of light revealing wounded men on stretchers and grasping tree branches along the narrow forest road.

The batteries powering the light bulbs began to run low, so the medical orderlies set up lamps with reflectors in the corners of the bandaging tent.

No more trucks arrived overnight, and by the morning the doctors managed to help everyone who had come to the medical battalion the previous day.

The battalion commander Svechnikov, in an undershirt and wide trousers, was sitting on the grass near the operating tent. He rubbed his hands slowly with his long, thin fingers. He was listening to Yezhov, who had sat down nearby with a notebook in his hands: 'One hundred and eighty-seven of one hundred and eighty-nine casualties were treated.'

'Two of them died, didn't they? Why?' the battalion commander asked, annoyed.

'Yes, two,' Yezhov sighed in distress and wiped his forehead with a handkerchief. 'Both had abdominal wounds and severe blood loss. The transfusion did not do any good. Also, a German was brought in, so Fadeev had to deal with him for more than two hours. If they had been sent to him right away...'

'Where's the prisoner now?' Svechnikov interrupted Yezhov.

'An employee of the special department came, and they took him away in a car. Maybe to divisional headquarters.'

'They must have needed him badly. Alright, go on.'

'We evacuated the lightly wounded, one hundred and

six, to the army field hospital. Two with jaw wounds and ten with craniocerebral wounds. Sixty-one are here. They are in the therapeutic, shock, and additional tents.'

'Provide care and control. And no more corpses!'

The executive officer walked off in the direction of the therapeutic tent, and Svechnikov sank down onto the grass and plunged into a deep sleep. Skvortsov, who was passing by with a canteen in his hand, looked at the sleeping battalion commander, shook his head with disapproval and dove into the ambulatory tent.

A minute later, he returned to Svechnikov and, carefully raising him a little, put a blanket and a pillow under his head and back. Then he took off his coat and covered the commander with it.

The thunder of the artillery bombardment woke the medical battalion and the patients, just as the sun had dried the morning dew from the grass and leaves of the shrubs.

'Today we'll begin later, probably yesterday was a particularly difficult day,' Nikolayenko said. After the morning routine, the whole platoon sat around eating barley porridge with canned meat in the open air.

Emptying her pot, Nikolayenko patted Antonina on the shoulder.

'Congratulations on your baptism of fire! You passed the test and didn't lag behind.'

Antonina glanced at Galina with confusion and said, 'What is there to say! I nearly passed out at the peak of the action.'

'First of all, "nearly" doesn't mean anything,' Galina

objected. 'I also passed out my first time, and so did the others. No need to dwell on it.'

Turning to her subordinates sitting nearby she loudly commanded, 'Time to put those calories to work. Fall in, ranks of two!'

'Comrade Doctor,' the senior orderly entreated, his voice betraying his disappointment, 'Can't we have a smoke?'

'Granted, anyone who is against fresh air can have a smoke. You've got five minutes,' Nikolayenko agreed.

She squatted a couple of times, turned to Antonina and said, 'From now on you can operate on your own. You're a bright young woman, and I see you're learning well on the fly. If there are any troubles, Katya or I will help you.'

'You, Galina, have golden hands. Where did you study?' Antonina asked with some admiration.

'In Moscow. I graduated from the First Medical Institute in 1939. I was sent to Gomel. There, I worked as a therapist in a clinic for two years. When the war began, I asked to be sent to the front. First I was in Bryansk, then in Kalinin. I've been here since January.'

She picked up two mess tins that had been left by the smokers and banged them against one another. Then she addressed the platoon, standing in two ranks: 'Check the state of the operating stations. The senior nurse will supply anything that's missing. The senior orderly will organize the washing and disinfection of the smocks and surgical coats, sheets, pillow-cases, and previously used bandaging material. Dismissed!'

'We have two and a half hours. I think we'll be ready' the battalion commander said to Antonina. 'Let's go to the bandaging tent.'

As it turned out, the wounded began to arrive much earlier. An hour after the preliminary bombardment had finished, a medical battalion truck brought the first group of twelve.

The escort, a senior medical assistant from the nearest regimental medical point, handed over some documents and reported, 'There are only badly wounded, all stretcher cases, with shrapnel wounds. Our troops began to attack, the fascists threw grenades and counterattacked. They almost managed to penetrate to our trenches. This man helped,' the assistant pointed at the first stretcher, placed on the grass. 'He replaced the machine gunner, who'd been killed, and drove the fascists away. And then a mortar landed in his trench. His left leg is in a bad state.'

'The surgeon will examine the case,' Letunov mumbled and signed the document confirming the arrival of the casualties. 'You are going back, aren't you?'

'Yes, I am. I'll bring the lightly wounded soldiers. There are about thirty of them.'

The first assistant jumped into the cab of the truck, and they drove off in the direction of the front line, leaving behind a cloud of dust.

'We'll operate in two teams,' Nikolayenko said glancing over the people in the bandaging tent. 'Antonina and I will be the first crew, the second team is Fadeev and Rita. The commissar is still with the battalion commander in the headquarters tent. Everyone else, carry on as before.'

The stretcher-bearers brought a casualty into the bandaging tent.

'Over here!' the platoon commander called, and pointed at the table in front of her.

'What's the matter with him?'

'Here you are, Comrade Doctor,' the orderly said, and handed the medical card to Nikolayenko.

Galina dismissed the orderly, read the wound description off the card and gave it to the senior nurse.

'File it away with the other new arrivals and prepare him for operating,' she said.

Looking at Antonina, she continued anxiously, 'We'll have to amputate the leg above the knee. The bone is broken and'

'Galina Petrovna!' the excited voice of Katerina interrupted Nikolayenko.

The senior nurse handed the medical card to Galina and pointed at something. Nikolayenro went pale, walked over to the stretcher and looked closely at the wounded man's face.

'It can't be! Katya, help me take off his tunic!' Nikolayenko said, extremely surprised.

Antonina didn't understand what was afoot. She watched the movements of the platoon commander and the nurse.

'Yes, it's him. Here's the wound in the shoulder. Almost no spots on the bandage. So, he did run away from us to the front after all,' Galina said, and shook her head.

It all dawned on Antonina just then: the soldier lying on the table was Sizov. He was the one who had disappeared the day before. He was the one with the self-inflicted wound.

'Let's get to work, girls,' Galina said, and quickly cut the left leg off his trousers to examine the wound.

'Urgent amputation! Prep him. I'll be in the sterilizing tent. Although…just prep him, quickly.'

Nikolayenko quickly left the bandaging tent and rushed to the headquarters.

'Amputation? A private? Sizov?' the battalion commissar responded in surprise once the breathless Nikolayenko had reported to him. 'Division Headquarters just phoned and asked about him.'

'What for?' Galina exclaimed.

'He was recommended for a decoration, the "For Courage" medal. They wanted to know how he is doing,' the commissar replied. 'They've nothing better to do at headquarters than phoning around,' he continued. 'We have to report to them immediately, you see. Where is Sizov now?'

'He is being prepared for operating.'

'Who will perform the operation?'

'I will, Matvey Ivanovich, it's just…' Galina stopped talking for a moment and then, troubled, she went on, 'I, as you know, perform guillotine amputations, and the boy is only eighteen. It would be better to give him an artificial limb, rather than end up with him on crutches.'

'Understood. Let's go.'

The commissar and Nikolayenko headed to the exit. Pirogov went to the sterilizing tent after examining the wounded soldier.

Galina whispered to Antonina, 'Your hands are already disinfected for operating, so you can assist Pirogov. Remember everything and watch carefully. He amputates according to the method of his great namesake.'

Antonina nodded in mute understanding. They could hear the sound of ambulance engines outside, again.

Lightning Source UK Ltd.
Milton Keynes UK
UKHW011819140622
404432UK00002B/51

9 781910 886946